Gluten-Free Mediterranean Diet Cookbook 2024

(Full-color Photo)

The Complete Easy and Healthy Everyday Mouthwatering Recipes without Gluten | No-Stress 7-Day Diet Meal Plan

Dr. SANDRA KAIN

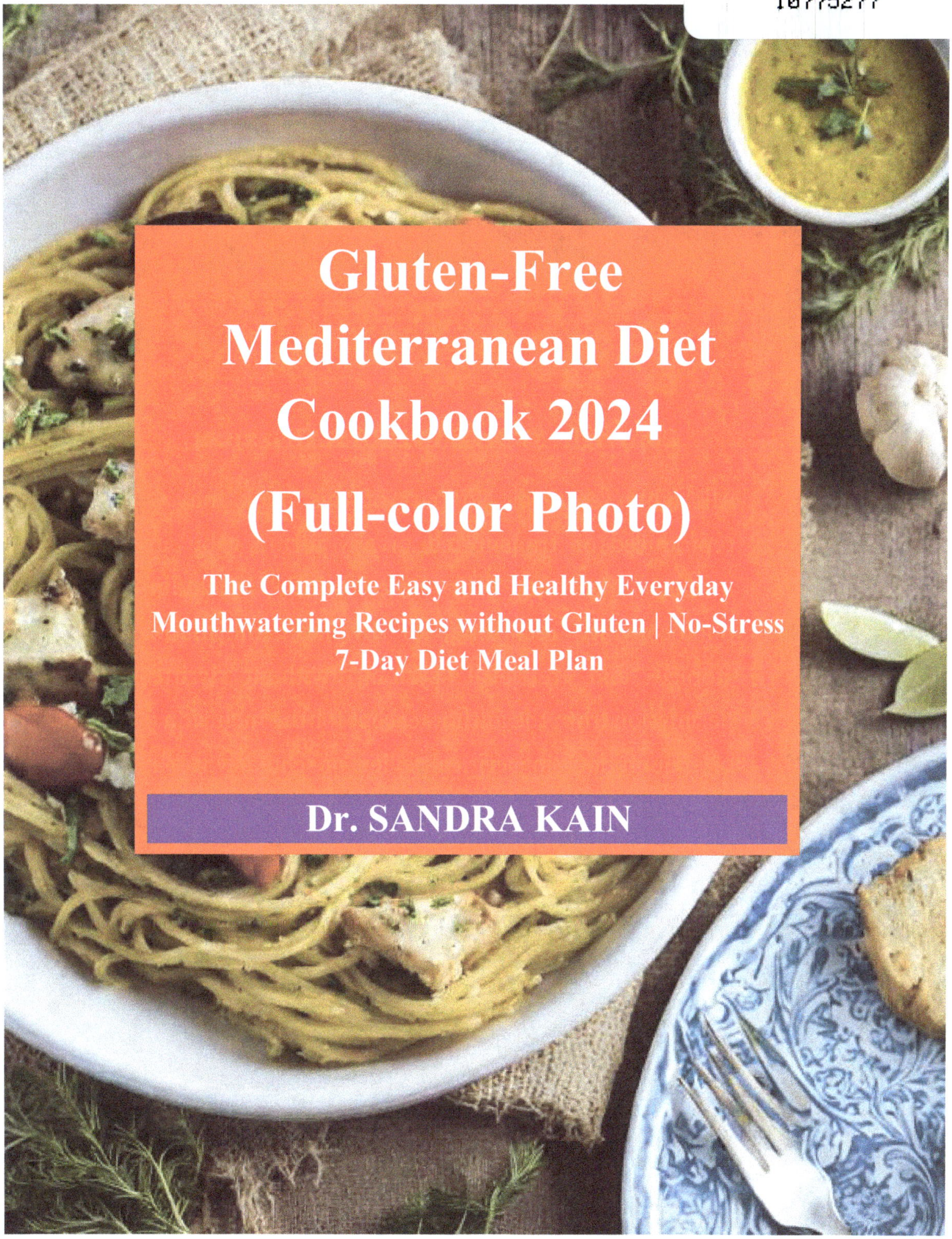

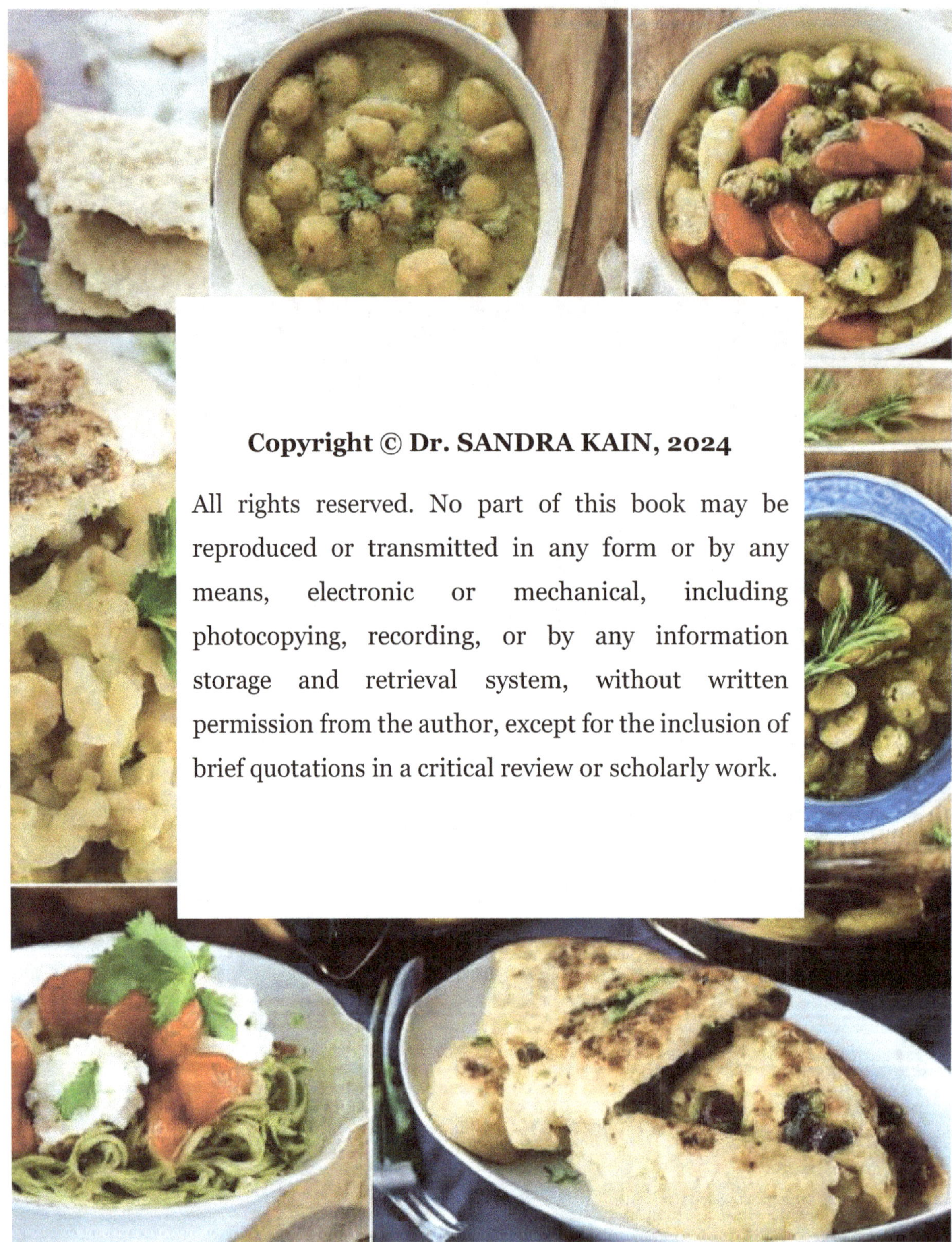

ABOUT THE AUTHOR

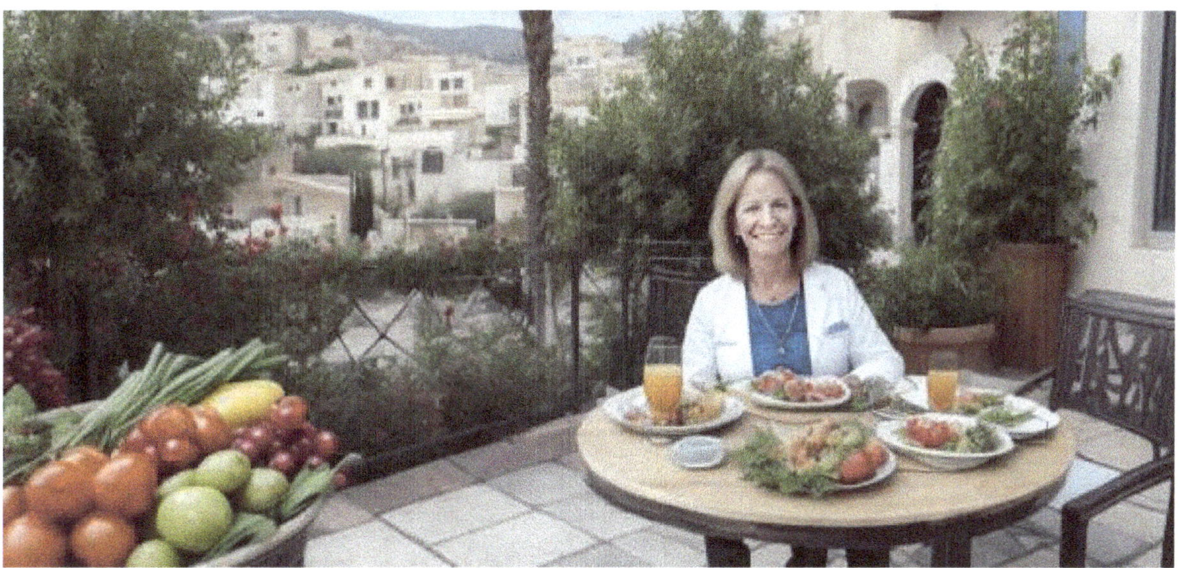

Dr. Sandra Kain isn't just a passionate cook and recipe developer; she's a doctor who understands the profound impact food has on our well-being. Her journey with the gluten-free Mediterranean diet began when she witnessed its transformative power in both her own life and the lives of her patients.

Driven by a desire to make this health-promoting lifestyle accessible to everyone, Dr. Kain embarked on a culinary mission. *"I wanted to show people that gluten-free doesn't have to mean bland or restrictive,"* she shares. *"The Mediterranean diet is a treasure trove of vibrant flavors, fresh ingredients, and nourishing goodness, and it translates beautifully to a gluten-free world."*

In "Gluten-Free Mediterranean Diet Cookbook," Dr. Kain offers more than just recipes; she provides a roadmap to a healthier, happier you. With **easy-to-follow, mouthwatering dishes,** she caters to a variety of dietary needs and preferences. Her **7-day meal plan** takes the guesswork out of gluten-free Mediterranean living, making it perfect for busy individuals and families alike.

Dr. Kain believes that cooking should be enjoyable, not stressful. Her recipes are designed with simplicity in mind, utilizing readily available ingredients and requiring minimal fuss. "I want people to find joy in the kitchen," she emphasizes. *"Cooking should be a celebration of flavor and togetherness, not a chore."*

Join Dr. Sandra Kain on a delicious adventure into the world of gluten-free Mediterranean cuisine. Discover how simple, healthy, and utterly satisfying eating can be with her vibrant recipes and practical tips. Let's raise a glass of (gluten-free, of course!) olive oil to enjoying flavorful food, vibrant health, and a life filled with culinary delights.

CONTENTS

INTRODUCTION

The Joys of Gluten-Free Mediterranean Cuisine

Imagine a beautiful place with sunny olive tree farms, a busy market where people talk and laugh, and yummy smells of herbs and garlic cooking. This is what the Mediterranean diet is all about - it's about enjoying tasty food with friends and family. The best part is, that you can still enjoy this delicious food even if you can't eat gluten. Gluten-free Mediterranean cooking is like a special key that opens the door to a world of healthy and yummy meals that will make your mouth water.

This is not a world where we have less of things, but a world where we can use our imagination. Instead of trying to find bread that doesn't have gluten, we can explore lots of different yummy foods like fruits, herbs, and special grains like quinoa and buckwheat. Instead of pancakes, we can make omelets with chickpea flour that are light and fluffy. Instead of pasta, we can enjoy delicious stews made with lentils. And instead of nuggets covered in breadcrumbs, we can have yummy roasted fish with a citrus glaze. This is not about being limited, but about being free to try new and exciting foods.

Unlocking the health benefits means finding out the good things that happen to our bodies when we do certain things. It's like discovering a secret treasure that makes us feel better and healthier. Discovering the positive effects on our well-being.

The Mediterranean diet is a really healthy way of eating that has been around for a long time. It's all about eating fresh and tasty foods, like fruits and vegetables, and using healthy fats in your meals. This diet can help protect your heart and prevent diseases like diabetes and cancer, and it can even be good for people who can't eat gluten.

Imagine eating foods that are good for your tummy, brain, and body. These foods have lots of fiber, healthy fats, and antioxidants. They help your body stay strong and healthy. You can enjoy them with your family and take your time to really enjoy the taste. It's also important to avoid processed foods and sugary snacks. Eating this way is not just about the food, but also about enjoying meals with the people you love and taking your time to cook.

Learning how to move around the kitchen with ease and without feeling scared or unsure.

Entering a gluten-free kitchen might seem scary at first, but don't worry! It's like going on an adventure where you can try new things. Instead of using regular flour, there are special flours like almond, coconut, and chickpea that make food taste different and have a different texture. You can make yummy sauces without using any animal products, and even make tasty tarts without a crust. You can also make delicious patties using lentils. It's about using your imagination and doing things you haven't done before!

This cookbook is like a special tool that helps you make yummy food. It tells you exactly what to do, gives you helpful tips, and has really cool recipes to try. It also explains important ingredients and how to use them and helps you plan meals easily if you can't eat gluten.

Get ready to explore a special kind of food that is good for your body and tastes yummy too! We are going on a fun journey to try out Mediterranean dishes that are gluten-free. It means they don't have a certain ingredient that some people can't eat. We will discover lots of tasty meals that make us feel happy and healthy. **Let's go on this adventure together and find new delicious foods to enjoy!**

Chapter 1: Gluten-Free Mediterranean Diet Foods & Shopping Grocery List

You are about to go on a pleasant journey through the tastes of the Mediterranean diet, but there is a delicious twist: it is an odyssey that does not include any gluten! Imagine that your kitchen has been turned into a sun-drenched port that is teeming with fresh produce, colorful spices, and heart-healthy foods, all of which are ready to be weaved into culinary magic. Instead of focusing on the taste, you should eliminate gluten, and be ready to chart your route toward a lifestyle that is both tasty and healthful.

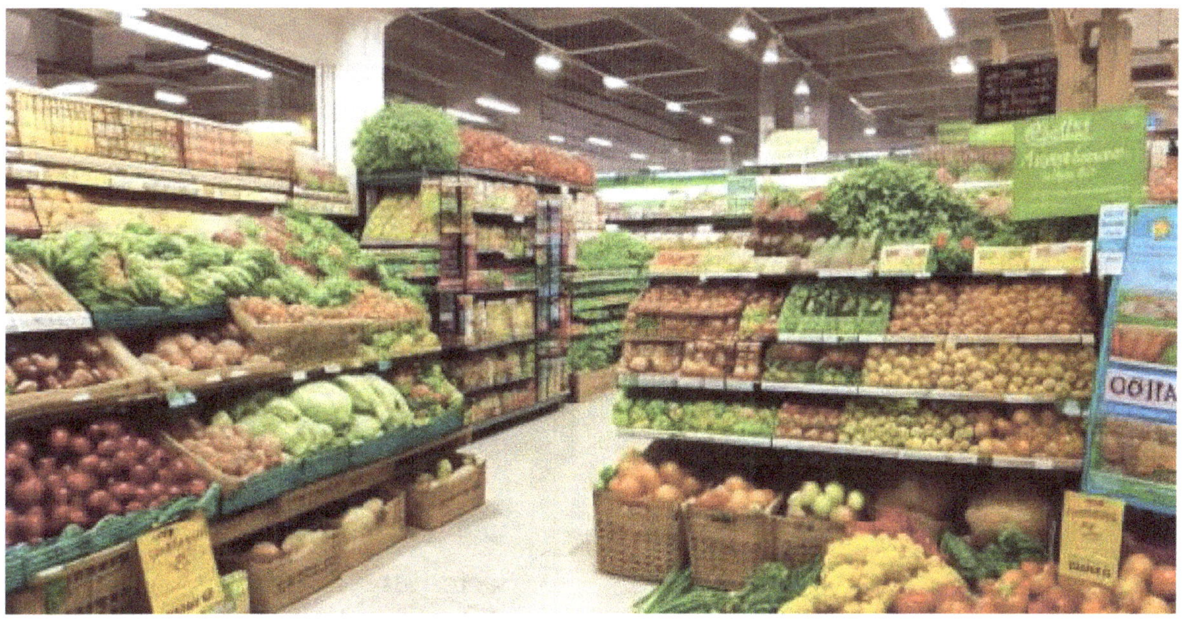

Prepare Your Pantry: An Emporium of Mediterranean Delights Awaits You Today

Imagine that you are at a lively marketplace in the Mediterranean region and go inside your pantry. Fruits and vegetables that have been matured by the sun are bursting out of their containers, presenting a rainbow of options. Be sure to stock up on these colorful jewels:

Fruits: Berries that turn your morning yogurt purple and crimson, citrus fruits that sing with the tangy heat of the sun, and seasonal delicacies such as peaches, figs, and melons that are just waiting to be converted into energizing compotes or fragrant sweets. Keep in mind that each new season brings with it fresh blessings to take pleasure in!

Vegetables: A Mediterranean tapestry: tomatoes blazing red, cucumbers cold and refreshing, peppers flaming with green and orange, leafy greens lending emerald brilliance, and the earthy depth of eggplant and mushrooms. They are the multi-talented heroes of your adventure through the world of cuisine.

Gluten-Free Grains: Forget tasteless crackers and uninspiring spaghetti! Quinoa, brown rice, millet, buckwheat, and gluten-free oats are your new pantry heroes. Imagine quinoa meals exploding with color, fluffy gluten-free pancakes, and lentil noodles whirling with brilliant sauces. Each grain gives a distinct texture and taste, eager to be discovered.

Healthy Fats: Extra virgin olive oil, your liquid gold, drizzles richness, and heart-healthy advantages on every meal. Don't forget about the pleasant textures and tastes of nuts, seeds, and olives. Their crunch and taste will add depth and texture to your recipes.

Protein Power: Build and sustain your power with the riches of the sea and land. Lean proteins like fish, poultry, and beans give sustainable energy, while lentils and tofu provide plant-based options rich in protein and fiber.

Dairy Delights: Yogurt, feta cheese, and goat cheese offer tangy undertones and calcium to your meals. Opt for lactose-free versions if required, assuring creamy richness without compromise.

Herbs & Spices: These are the fragrant alchemists who convert ordinary items into gourmet wonders. Let fresh herbs like basil, oregano, and thyme weave their aromatic charms. Don't forget about spices like cumin, paprika, and turmeric, their warm fragrances and powerful tastes are ready to stimulate your taste senses.

Beyond the Basics: Venturing into Uncharted Territory

Your Mediterranean adventure doesn't finish at the cost of your pantry essentials. Discover secret gems that will enhance your gastronomic horizons:

Gluten-Free Breads and Pastas: Forget gluten-free bread that crumbles like sand! Explore the world of bread made from rice, almond, or coconut flour, each giving a distinct texture and taste. Brown rice or lentil pasta are wonderful options, ready to be tossed with your favorite sauces.

Ancient Grains: Amaranth, sorghum, and teff are the seasoned captains of the grain world, bringing distinct tastes and outstanding nutritional profiles. These ancient grains will give depth and texture to your dishes, from hearty morning porridge to fluffy gluten-free bread.

Plant-Based Milk: Unsweetened almond, coconut, or oat milk is wonderful for smoothies, coffee, and cereal, bringing their creamy richness without the gluten. Imagine a morning smoothie overflowing with berries and mixed with almond milk, or a cozy dish of oatmeal drenched in creamy coconut milk.

Olives & Tapenades: These briny pleasures are the naughty pirates of your culinary landscape, giving a punch of flavor to salads, sandwiches, and roasted veggies. Whether you love plump Kalamata olives or explore the world of tapenades, they'll provide a welcome blast of zest to your meal.

Remember, Your Journey Needs a Map:

Label Sleuth: Be a detective! Hidden gluten may be hidden in processed foods. Always examine labels carefully, ensuring sure items are certified gluten-free.

Variety Voyage: The Mediterranean diet is a kaleidoscope of tastes and sensations. Experiment with new ingredients and recipes to keep your dinners intriguing. Don't be afraid to try new fruits and vegetables, explore various herbs and spices, and tinker with culinary methods.

Home Cook Hero: Take the helm of your kitchen! Cooking at home provides you control over ingredients and portion proportions. Learn fundamental culinary skills, and master easy recipes, and soon you'll be churning up Mediterranean delicacies with confidence.

Savor the Journey: The Mediterranean diet is not a sprint, it's a marathon of good living. Savor the tastes of fresh ingredients, enjoy the act of a profile picture continue creating from where you stop cooking, and rejoice in the beneficial influence on your health. This is a lifestyle to embrace, not a short diet to tolerate.

Adventure Awaits: Embrace the Mediterranean Spirit

Embracing a gluten-free Mediterranean diet is more than simply a change in food; it's a transformation in thinking. Embrace the following concepts to make this trip really transformative:

Slow Down and Savor: Meals are not simply about nourishment; they're occasions for connection and pleasure. Slow down, taste each mouthful, and cherish the companionship of loved ones.

Honor the Seasons: Celebrate the wealth of fresh food by picking fruits and vegetables at their best. Let the seasons dictate your cuisine and indulge in the ever-changing tastes.

Embrace Freshness: Prioritize whole, raw foods above packaged items. Fill your kitchen with vivid items that fuel your body and stimulate your senses.

Cook with Love: Infuse your cuisine with passion and creativity. Let cooking be a thoughtful activity, a method to demonstrate your caring for yourself and others.

Share the Bounty: Gather around the table with friends and family, exchanging tales and laughing as you break bread together. Food is designed to be eaten in company, encouraging connection and pleasure.

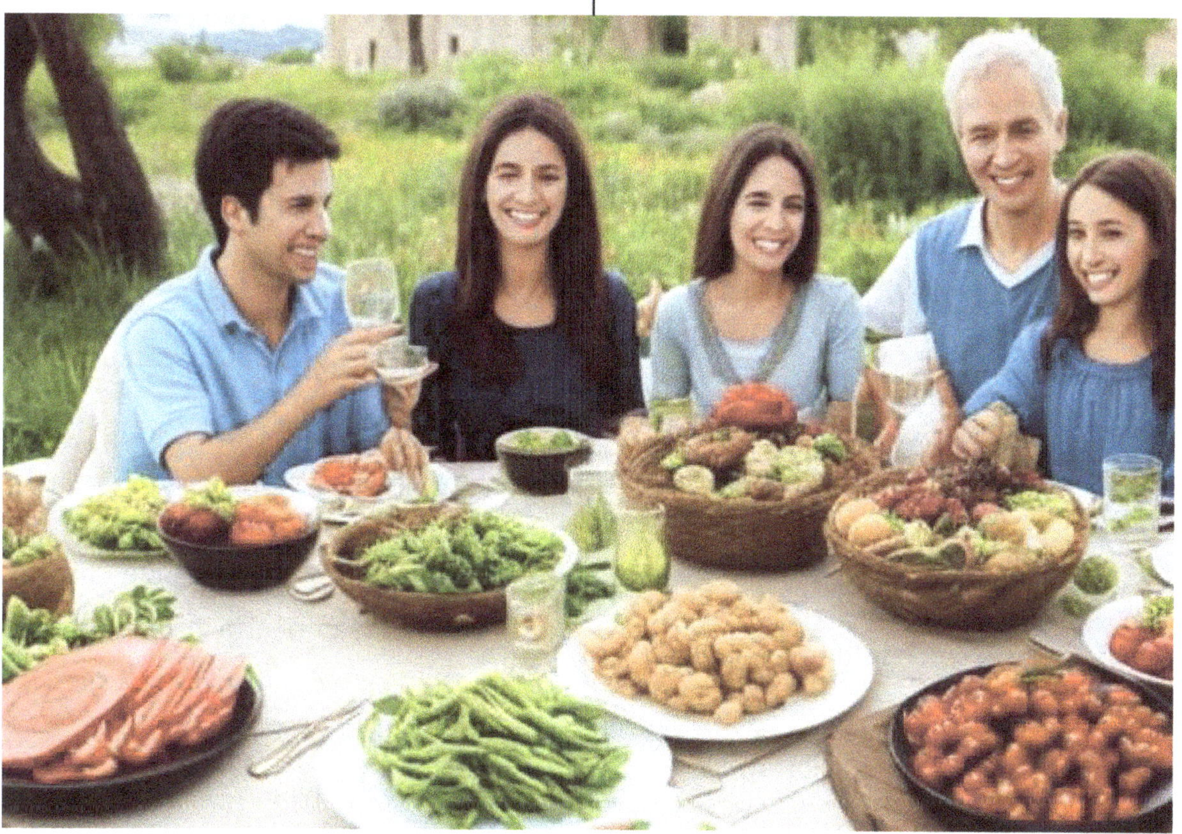

Set Sail on Your Gluten-Free Mediterranean Odyssey

The Mediterranean diet, with its concentration on fresh, tasty products, works nicely with a gluten-free lifestyle. Embrace this voyage, and you'll find a world of colorful foods, strong health, and a newfound appreciation for the simple joys of delicious food, shared meals, and a life well-lived. Bon voyage, and may your trip be full of delightful discoveries!

Chapter 2: Breakfast Recipes

Mediterranean Breakfast Bruschetta

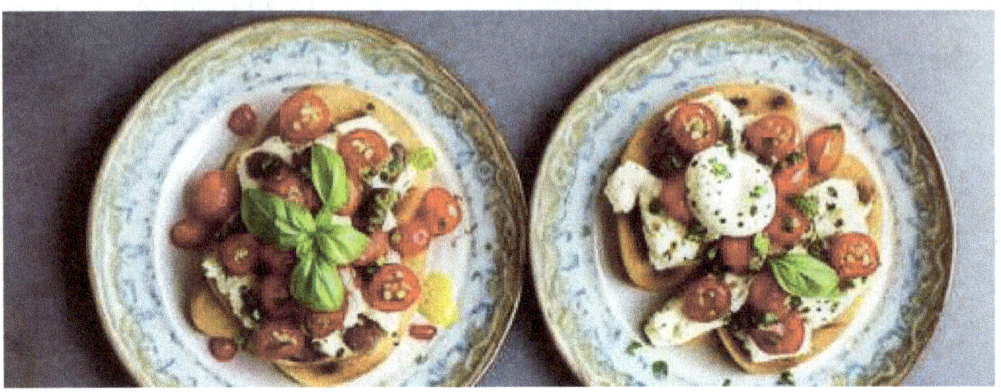

Prep Time: 5 minutes	
Cooking Time: 10 minutes (if grilling tomatoes)	
Total Time: 15 minutes	
Serving: 1 piece of toast	

Ingredients:

- 1 slice of gluten-free multigrain bread
- 2 tablespoons ricotta cheese
- 2-3 sun-dried tomatoes or 1-2 grilled tomatoes, sliced 5 Kalamata olives, halved
- Drizzle of olive oil
- Pinch of fresh thyme

Directions:

1. Toast bread till golden brown.
2. Spread ricotta cheese on bread.
3. Top with tomato slices, olives, olive oil drizzle, and sprinkle with thyme.

Nutritional Information: (approximate per serving)

Calories: 250 | Fat: 12g | Carbohydrates: 28g | Protein: 10g

Shakshuka with Sweet Potato Hash

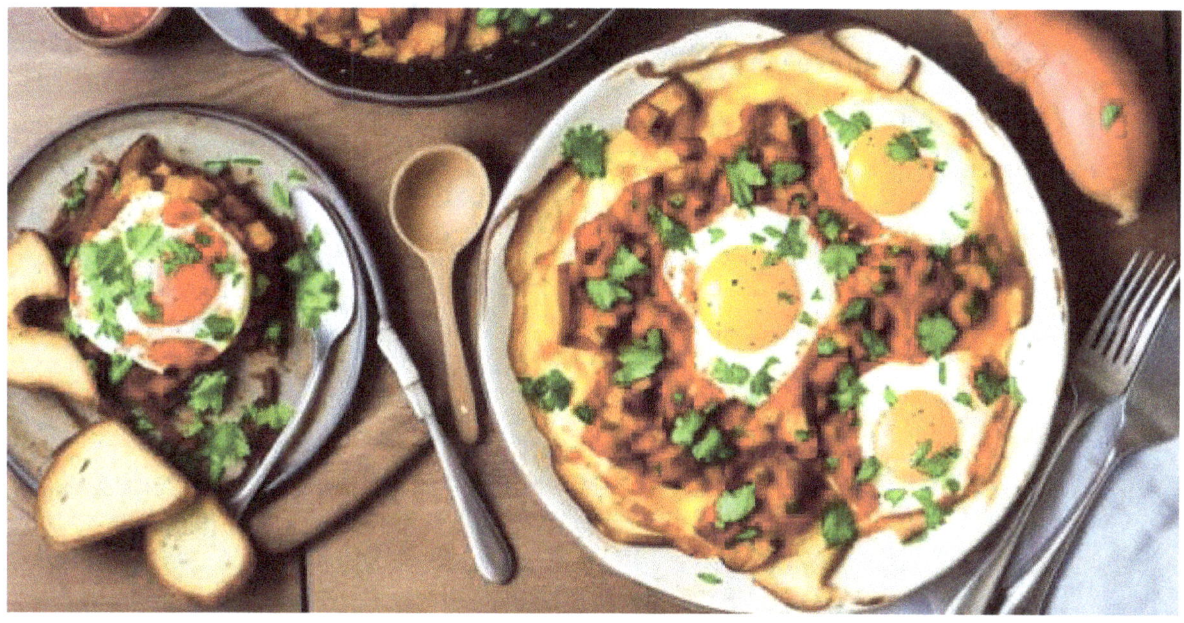

Prep Time: 10 minutes	
Cooking Time: 20-25 minutes	
Total Time: 30-35 minutes	
Serving: 1-2 persons	

Ingredients:

- 1 medium sweet potato, diced
- 1/2 onion, chopped
- 1 bell pepper, chopped
- 1 tablespoon olive oil
- 1/2 teaspoon cumin
- 1/4 teaspoon paprika
- Salt and pepper to taste
- 2 eggs
- Gluten-free toast or pita bread (optional)

Directions:

1. Saute sweet potato, onion, and pepper in olive oil until tender.

2. Season with cumin, paprika, salt, and pepper.
3. Create wells in the mixture and break an egg into each.
4. Bake at 400°F (200°C) for 10-12 minutes, or until egg whites are set.

5. You can eat this food with either toast or pita bread and dip it in the sauce.

Nutritional Information: (approximate per serving with 1 egg)

Calories: 350 | Fat: 15g | Carbohydrates: 35g | Protein: 15g

Coconut Chia Seed Pudding with Berries and Pistachios

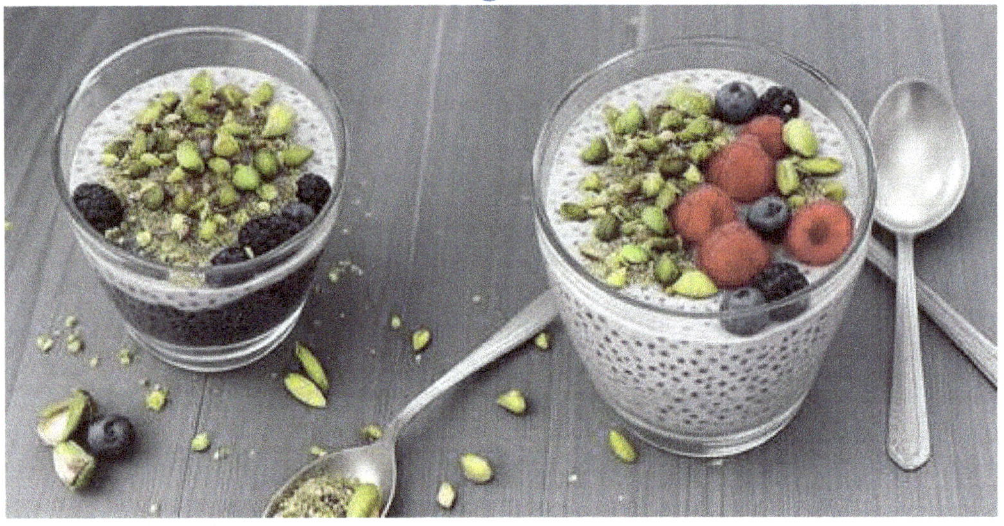

Prep Time: 5 minutes (including overnight soaking)
Cooking Time: 0
Total Time: 10 minutes (including overnight soaking)
Serving: 1 jar

Ingredients:

- 1/4 cup chia seeds
- 1 cup unsweetened coconut milk
- 1 tablespoon honey
- 1/2 teaspoon vanilla extract
- 1/2 cup fresh berries
- 1/4 cup chopped pistachios
- 1 tablespoon Greek yogurt (optional)

Directions:

1. Combine chia seeds, coconut milk, honey, and vanilla essence in a container. Stir thoroughly and chill overnight.
2. In the morning, top with berries, pistachios, and yogurt (if using).

Nutritional Information: (approximate per serving without yogurt)

Calories: 250 | Fat: 15g | Carbohydrates: 25g | Protein: 5g

Baked Frittata Muffins with Spinach and Feta:

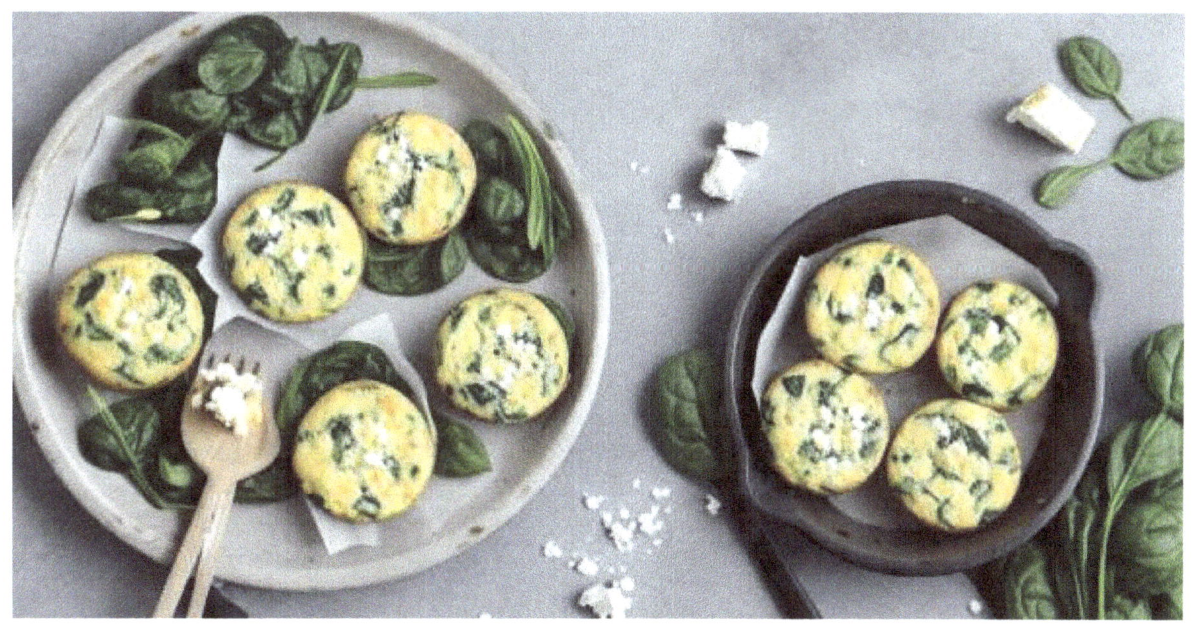

| Prep Time: 10 minutes |
| Cooking Time: 20-25 minutes |
| Total Time: 30-35 minutes |
| Serving: 6-8 muffins |

Ingredients:

- 4 eggs
- 1/2 cup chopped spinach
- 1/4 cup crumbled feta cheese
- 1/4 cup chopped onion
- 1/4 teaspoon dried oregano
- Salt and pepper to taste
- Olive oil spray

Directions:

1. Preheat oven to 375°F (190°C).
2. Whisk eggs in a bowl. Stir in spinach, feta cheese, onion, oregano, salt, and pepper.
3. Spray the muffin pan with olive oil and fill each cup with egg mixture.
4. Bake for 20-25 minutes, or until set.

Nutritional Information: (approximate per muffin)

Calories: 70, Fat: 5g , Carbohydrates: 1g, Protein: 5g

Spiced Chickpea Fritters with Yogurt Dip:

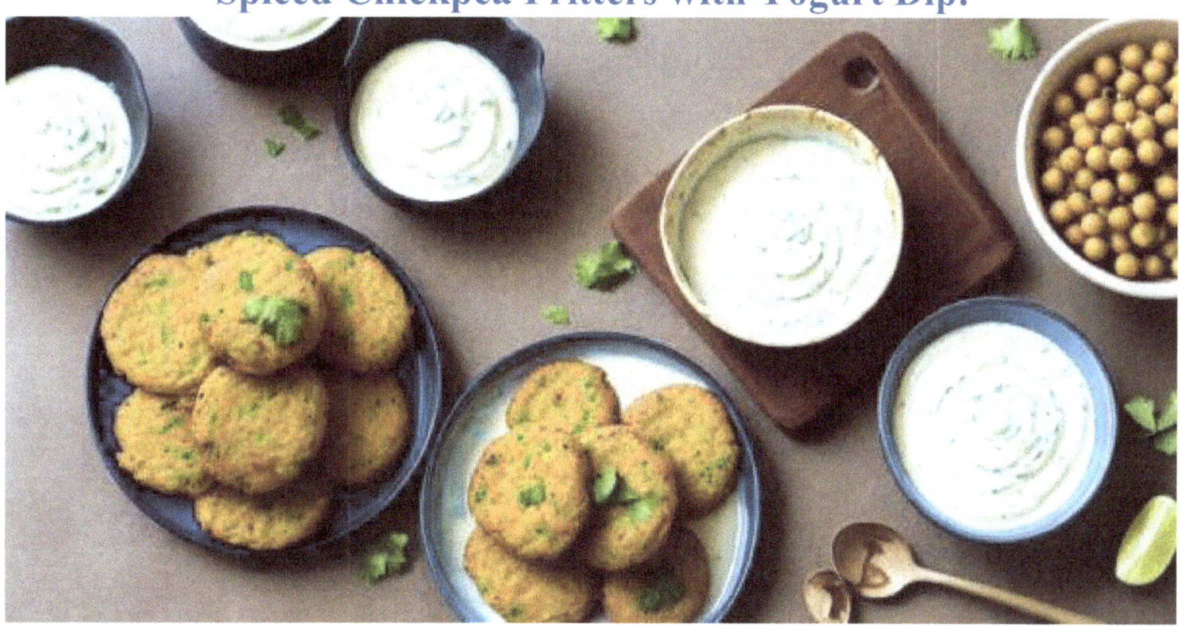

Prep Time: 15 minutes
Cooking Time: 10-15 minutes
Total Time: 25-30 minutes
Serving: 4 fritters

Ingredients:

- one can (15 ounces) of chickpeas, drained and rinsed
- 1/4 cup gluten-free flour (such as chickpea flour or brown rice flour)
- 1/4 cup chopped onion
- 1/4 cup chopped cilantro
- 1/2 teaspoon turmeric
- 1/2 teaspoon garam masala
- Salt and pepper to taste
- Olive oil for frying
- Cucumber yogurt dip: 1/2 cup Greek yogurt
- 1/2 cucumber, grated and drained
- 1/4 teaspoon dill
- Salt and pepper to taste

Directions:

1. Mash chickpeas in a bowl using a fork or potato masher.
2. Stir in flour, onion, cilantro, spices, salt, and pepper.
3. Form the ingredients into tiny patties.
4. Put oil in a pan and turn on the stove to medium heat.
5. Fry fritters for 3-4 minutes on each side, or until golden brown.
6. For the dip: Combine yogurt, cucumber, dill, salt, and pepper in a bowl.
7. Serve fritters with cucumber yogurt dip.

Nutritional Information: (approximate per fritter)

Calories: 150 | Fat: 5g | Carbohydrates: 20g | Protein: 8g

Chapter 3: Lunch Recipes

Greek Chicken Pita Salad Bowl:

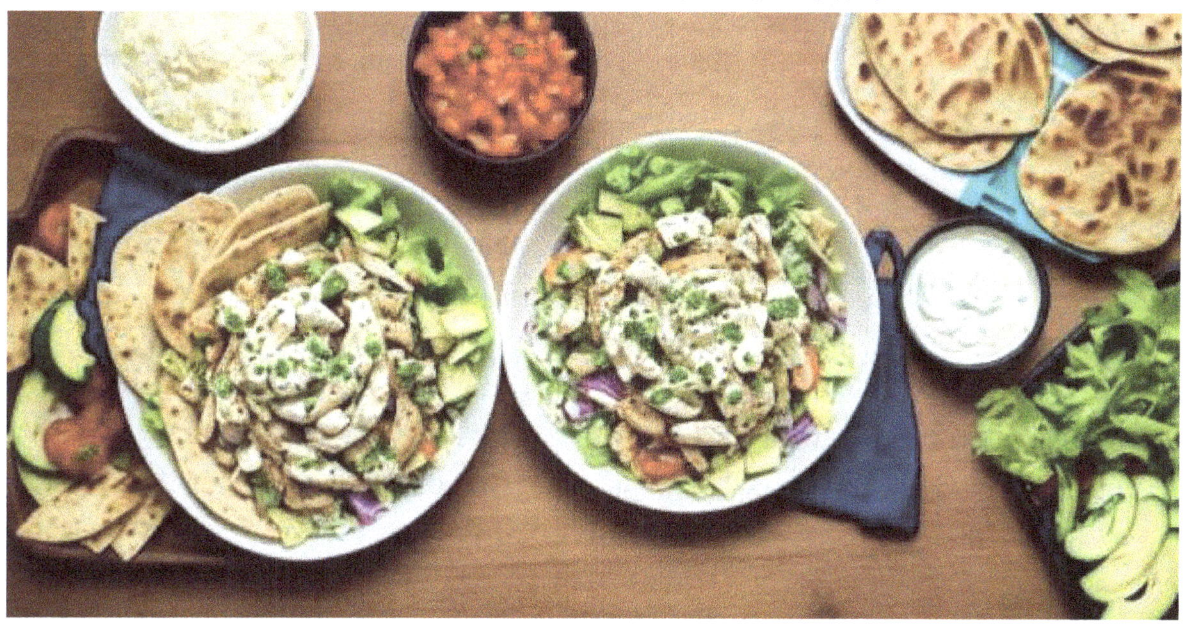

Prep Time: 15 minutes (including marinating time)	
Cooking Time: 20-25 minutes (depending on cooking technique)	
Total Time: 35-40 minutes	
Serving: 1 dish or pita bread	

Ingredients:

- 1 boneless, skinless chicken breast, sliced into bite-sized pieces
- 2 tablespoons olive oil
- 1 tablespoon lemon juice
- 1 teaspoon dried oregano
- 1/2 teaspoon garlic powder
- Salt and pepper to taste
- 2 cups chopped romaine lettuce
- 1/2 cucumber, chopped 1 tomato, chopped 1/4 cup Kalamata olives, halved
- 1/4 red onion, thinly sliced

- 1/4 cup crumbled feta cheese
- Vinaigrette dressing of your choosing (olive oil and vinegar, balsamic vinaigrette, etc.)
- Gluten-free pita bread (optional)

Directions:

1. Marinate chicken in olive oil, lemon juice, oregano, garlic powder, salt, and pepper for at least 30 minutes.
2. Grill or bake chicken until cooked through (internal temp 165°F).
3. Combine lettuce, cucumber, tomato, olives, red onion, and feta cheese in a bowl.
4. Add cooked chicken and sprinkle with vinaigrette dressing.
5. Serve in a dish or wrap in gluten-free pita bread.

Nutritional Information: (approximate per serving)

Calories: 400-500 (depending on dressing and pita bread) | Fat: 15-20g | Carbohydrates: 30-40g | Protein: 30-40g

Mediterranean Quinoa Tabbouleh:

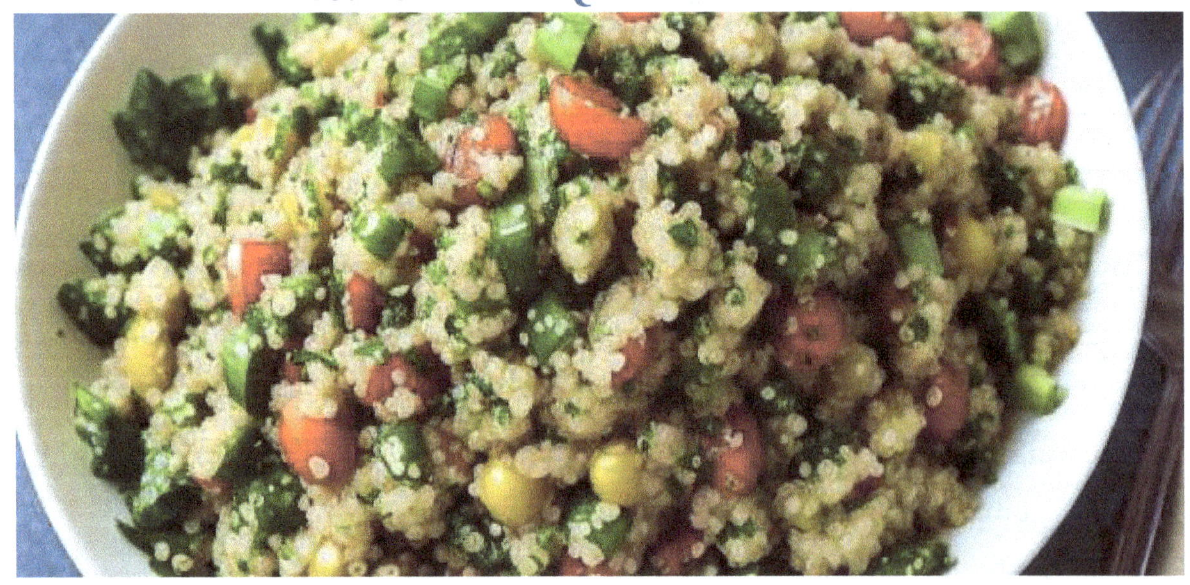

Prep Time: 10 minutes
Cooking Time: 15 minutes
Total Time: 25 minutes
Serving: 2-3 persons

Ingredients:

- 1 cup quinoa, washed
- 1 1/2 cups chopped parsley
- 1/2 cup chopped mint
- 1 tomato, chopped 1 cucumber, chopped 1/4 cup scallions, chopped 2 tablespoons olive oil
- 1 tablespoon lemon juice
- Salt and pepper to taste
- Optional: Chickpeas or lentils (cooked), for extra protein

Directions:

1. Cook quinoa according per package directions.
2. Combine cooked quinoa, parsley, mint, tomato, cucumber, and scallions in a bowl.
3. Drizzle with olive oil and lemon juice. Season with salt and pepper.
4. Stir in cooked chickpeas or lentils (if using).
5. Serve refrigerated or at room temperature.

Nutritional Information: (approximate per serving)

Calories: 250-300 (depending on extra protein) | Fat: 10-15g | Carbohydrates: 35-40g | Protein: 8-15g (with chickpeas or lentils)

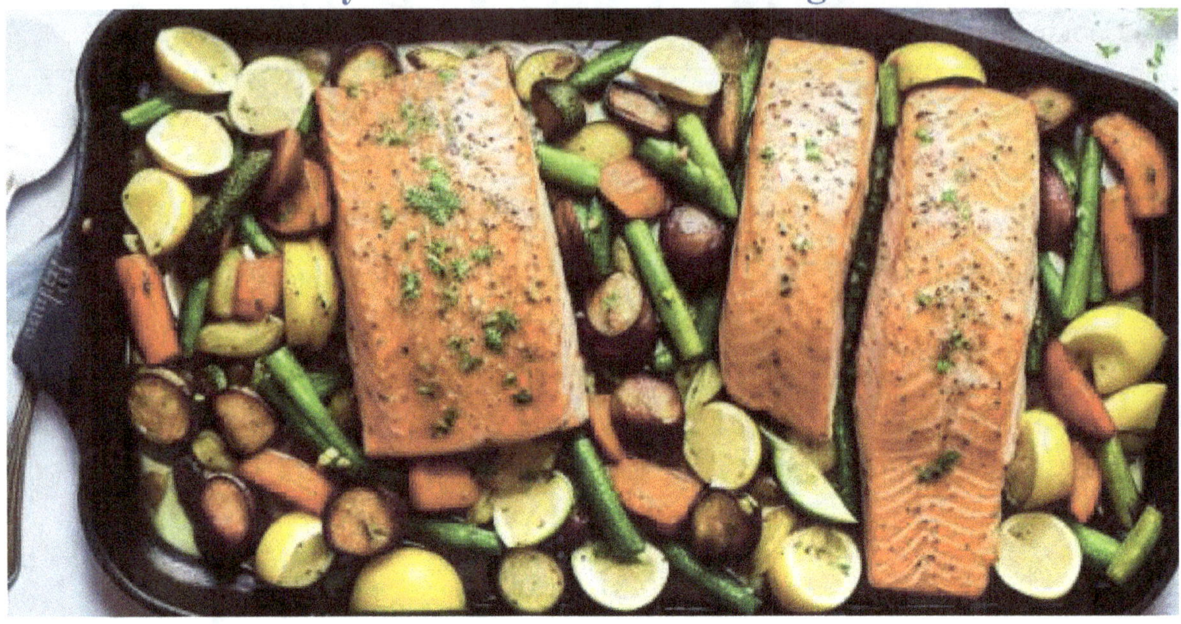

Prep Time: 10 minutes	
Cooking Time: 20-25 minutes	
Total Time: 30-35 minutes	
Serving: 1-2 persons	

Ingredients:

- 2 salmon fillets
- 1 tablespoon lemon juice
- 1 teaspoon dried oregano
- 1/2 teaspoon paprika
- Salt and pepper to taste
- 1 zucchini, chopped
- 1 bell pepper, chopped
- 1 red onion, chopped
- 1 tablespoon olive oil
- 1 tablespoon balsamic vinegar
- Brown rice, quinoa, or side salad (optional)

Directions:

1. Preheat oven to 400°F (200°C).
2. Season fish with lemon juice, oregano, paprika, salt, and pepper.

3. Toss zucchini, bell pepper, and red onion with olive oil and distribute on a baking sheet.

4. Place salmon fillets on top of veggies.

5. Roast for 20-25 minutes, or until salmon is cooked through and veggies are soft.

6. Drizzle with balsamic vinegar before serving.

7. Pair with brown rice, quinoa, or a side salad (optional).

Tuna Salad Lettuce Wraps:

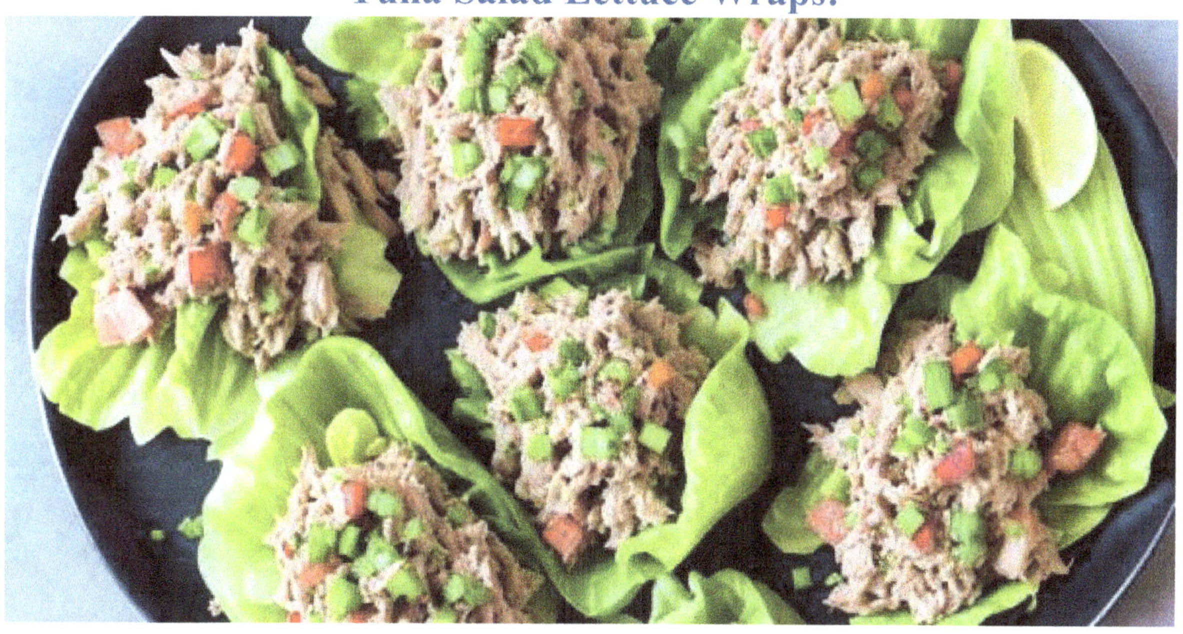

Prep Time: 10 minutes	
Total Time: 10 minutes	
Serving: 2 wraps	

Ingredients:

- 1 can (5 oz) tuna, drained
- 1/4 cup chopped celery
- 1/4 cup chopped red onion
- 2 teaspoons chopped fresh dill
- 2 tablespoons Greek yogurt or mayonnaise
- 1 tablespoon lemon juice
- Salt and pepper to taste
- 4 big romaine lettuce leaves
- 1/4 cup crumbled feta cheese
- Cherry tomatoes, halved (optional)

Directions:

1. Combine tuna, celery, red onion, dill, yogurt or mayonnaise, lemon juice, salt, and pepper in a bowl.
2. Fill each lettuce leaf with tuna salad.
3. Top with feta cheese and cherry tomatoes (if using).

Nutritional Information: (approximate per wrap)

Calories: 250 | Fat: 10g | Carbohydrates: 15g | Protein: 25g

Chickpea Falafel Salad Sandwich:

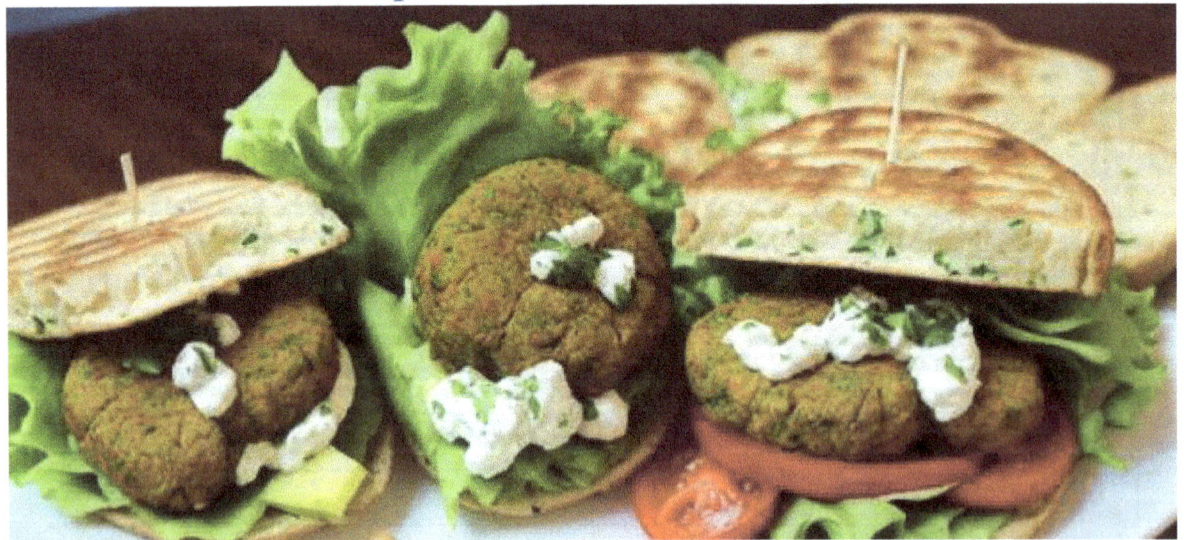

Prep Time: 15 minutes
Cooking Time: 20-25 minutes
Total Time: 35-40 minutes
Serving: 2 sandwiches

Ingredients:

- one can (15 ounce) of chickpeas, drained and rinsed
- 1/2 onion, chopped
- 1/4 cup chopped parsley
- 1/4 cup cilantro
- 2 cloves garlic, minced
- 1 teaspoon cumin
- 1/2 teaspoon coriander
- Salt and pepper to taste
- 1/4 cup gluten-free flour (such as chickpea flour or brown rice flour)
- Olive oil for frying
- 2 gluten-free pita breads or 4 big lettuce leaves
- 1 tomato, chopped
- 1/2 cucumber, chopped
- 1/4 red onion, thinly sliced
- Parsley leaves, for garnish
- Tahini sauce, for serving

Directions:

1. Preheat oven to 400°F (200°C).
2. In a food processor, blend chickpeas, onion, parsley, cilantro, garlic, cumin, coriander, salt, and pepper. Pulse until coarsely crushed.
3. Transfer mixture to a bowl and whisk in flour.
4. Shape ingredients into tiny patties.
5. In a skillet, heat the oil over medium heat.
6. Fry falafel for 2-3 minutes each side, or until golden brown.
7. Transfer falafel to a baking sheet and bake for 10-15 minutes, or until cooked through.
8. Fill pita breads or lettuce leaves with falafel, veggies, parsley, and tahini sauce.

Nutritional Information: (approximate per sandwich)

Calories: 450-500 (depending on pita bread) | Fat: 15-20g | Carbohydrates: 60-70g | Protein: 20-25g

One-Pan Lemon Garlic Cod with Roasted Vegetables

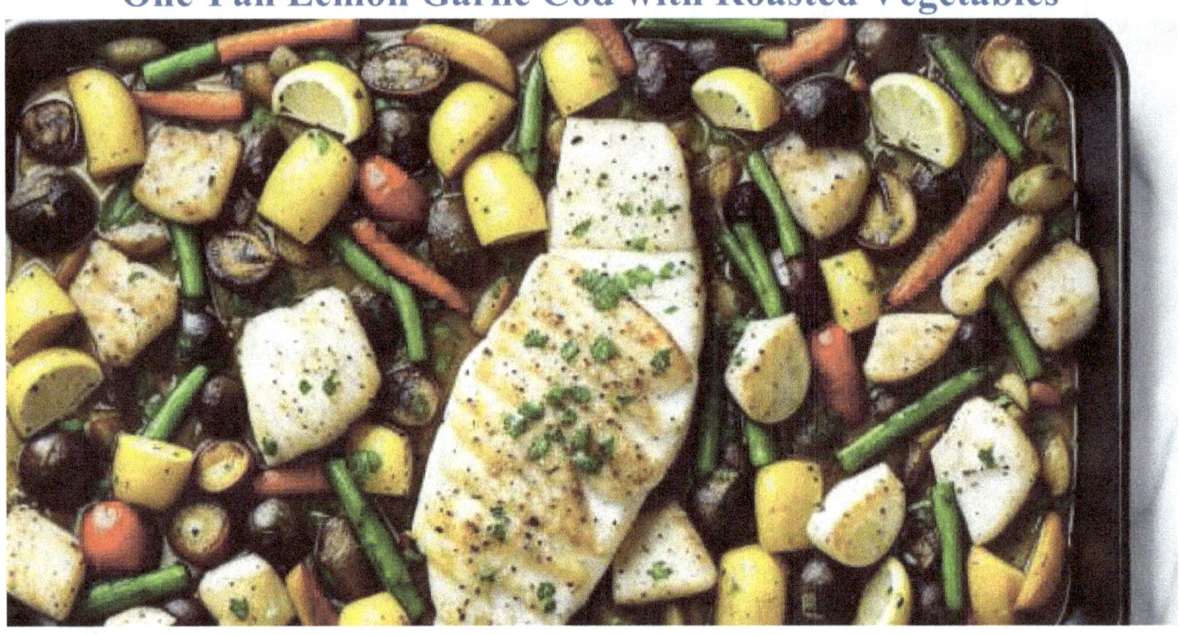

Prep Time: 10 minutes	
Cooking Time: 25-30 minutes	
Total Time: 35-40 minutes	
Serving: 2-3 persons	

Ingredients:

- 2 medium zucchini, sliced
- 2 yellow squash, sliced
- 1 cup cherry tomatoes
- 2 tablespoons olive oil
- 1 teaspoon dried oregano
- 1/2 teaspoon garlic powder
- Salt and pepper to taste
- 2 fish fillets (approximately 6 oz each)
- 1 tablespoon lemon juice
- Fresh parsley, chopped (optional)

Directions:

1. Preheat oven to 400°F (200°C).

2. Toss zucchini, squash, and tomatoes with olive oil, oregano, garlic powder, salt, and pepper. Spread on a baking sheet.

3. Season fish fillets with salt and pepper. Lay on top of veggies.

4. Roast for 25-30 minutes, or until fish is flaky and veggies are soft.

5. Squeeze some lemon juice on top and sprinkle parsley over it before you eat it.

Nutritional Information: (approximate per serving)

Calories: 400-500 | Fat: 15-20g | Carbohydrates: 40-50g | Protein: 30-35g

Grilled Haloumi Salad with Quinoa and Herbs

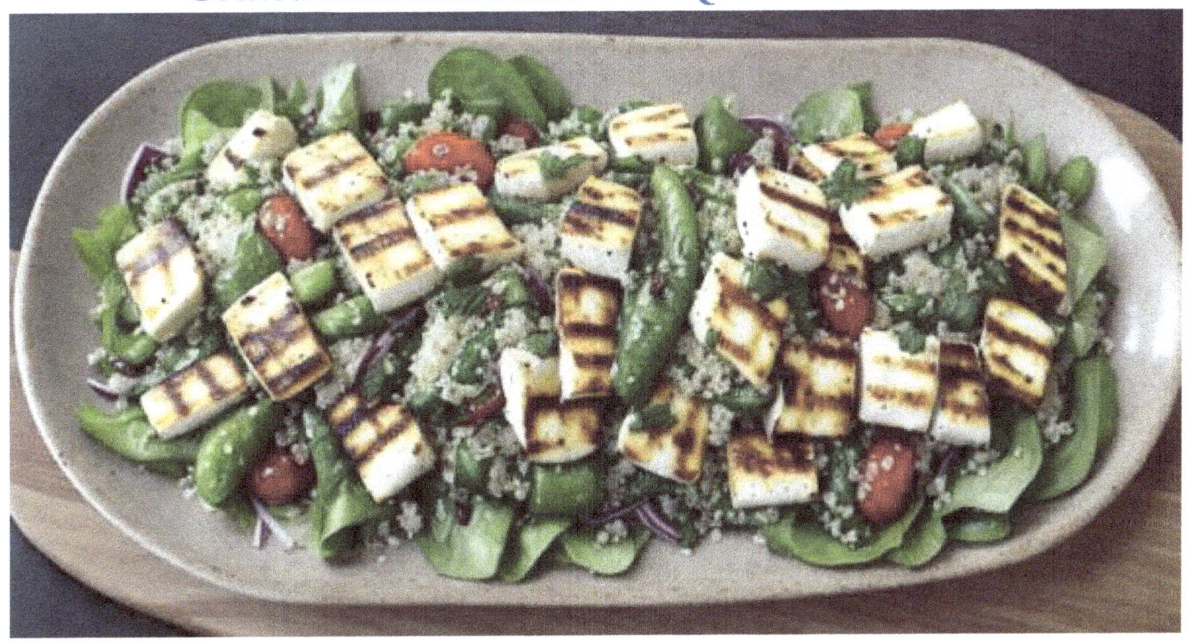

Prep Time: 15 minutes
Cooking Time: 10-15 minutes (plus quinoa cooking time)
Total Time: 25-30 minutes
Serving: 2-3 persons

Ingredients:

- 1 cup quinoa, washed
- 1 tablespoon olive oil
- 1/2 red onion, thinly sliced
- 1 tomato, chopped
- 1 cucumber, chopped
- 1/4 cup Kalamata olives, halved
- 1/4 red onion, thinly sliced
- 1/2 lemon, juiced
- 1 tablespoon olive oil
- 1 teaspoon dried oregano
- 1/2 teaspoon salt
- 1/4 teaspoon black pepper
- 1 (8 oz) package haloumi cheese, cut thick
- Fresh mint and oregano leaves, for garnish

Directions:

1. Cook quinoa according per package directions.
2. While quinoa cooks, make salad: Combine onion, tomato, cucumber, olives, and red onion in a bowl.
3. In a separate dish, combine lemon juice, olive oil, oregano, salt, and pepper.
4. Grill haloumi slices until golden brown on all sides.
5. Add cooked quinoa to salad dish and stir with dressing.
6. Top with grilled haloumi cheese and garnish with fresh mint and oregano.

Nutritional Information: (approximate per serving)

Calories: 450-500 | Fat: 15-20g | Carbohydrates: 50-60g | Protein: 20-25g

Baked Stuffed Peppers with Lentils & Herbs: A Flavorful Journey

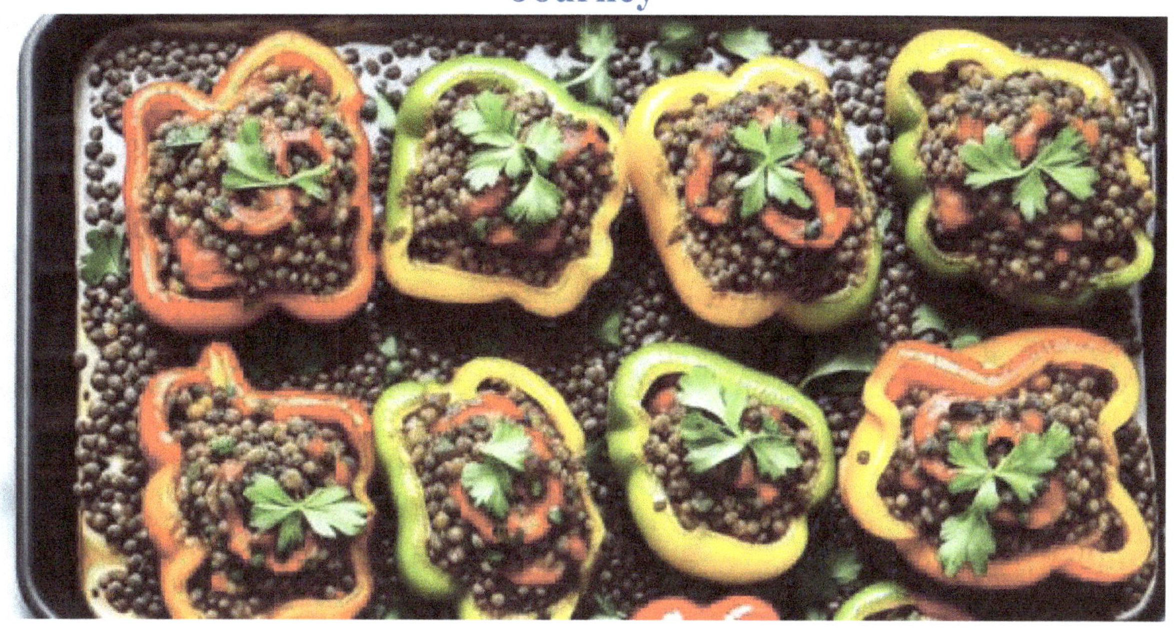

Prep Time: 20 minutes	
Cooking Time: 40-45 minutes	
Total Time: 60-65 minutes	
Serving: 4-6 persons	

Ingredients:

- 2 cups cooked lentils (or 1 cup dried lentils, washed and cooked according to package directions)
- 1 cup cooked brown rice
- 1 (15 oz) can chopped tomatoes, undrained
- 1/2 onion, chopped
- 2 cloves garlic, minced
- 1 teaspoon cumin
- 1/2 teaspoon paprika
- Salt and pepper to taste
- 4 bell peppers, halves and seeds removed

- 1/4 cup crumbled feta cheese Greek yogurt, for serving (optional)

Directions:

1. Preheat oven to 375°F (190°C).
2. In a large bowl, add cooked lentils, brown rice, chopped tomatoes, onion, garlic, cumin, paprika, salt, and pepper. Mix thoroughly to mix.
3. Fill each bell pepper half with the lentil mixture, packing it in carefully.
4. Place the filled peppers on a baking dish with the open side facing up.
5. Bake for 40-45 minutes, or until the peppers are soft and the mixture is cooked through.
6. Remove from the oven and top each pepper half with crumbled feta cheese.
7. Serve warm with a dollop of Greek yogurt, if preferred.

Nutritional Information (per serving):

Calories: 300-350 (depending on the size of the peppers and toppings) | Fat: 5-10g | Carbohydrates: 40-45g | Protein: 15-20g | Fiber: 5-10g

Shrimp Scampi with Zucchini Noodles:

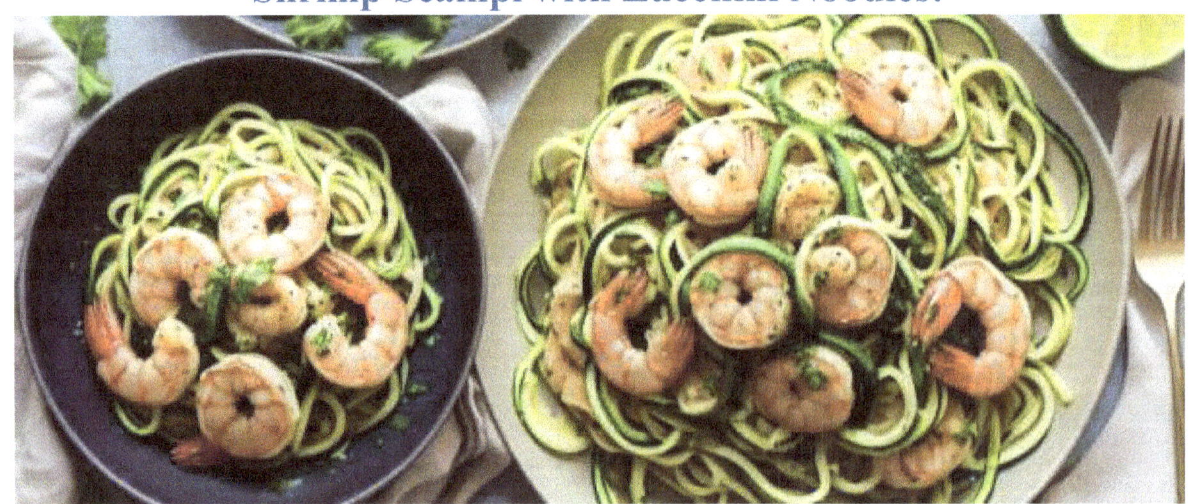

| Prep Time: 15 minutes |
| Cooking Time: 10-15 minutes |
| Total Time: 25-30 minutes |
| Serving: 2-3 persons |

Ingredients:

- 1-pound shrimp, peeled and deveined
- 2 tablespoons olive oil
- 4 cloves garlic, minced
- 1/4 teaspoon red pepper flakes
- 1/4 cup dry white wine
- 2 medium zucchini, spiralized into noodles
- 1 cup cherry tomatoes, halved
- 1/4 cup fresh basil leaves, chopped 1/2 lemon, juiced
- Salt and pepper to taste
- Parmesan cheese, grated (optional)

Directions:

1. Put olive oil in a big pan and turn the heat to medium.
2. Add garlic and red pepper flakes and sauté for 1 minute, until aromatic.
3. Add shrimp and cook for 2-3 minutes each side, or until pink and opaque.
4. Deglaze the pan with white wine, scraping out any browned pieces.
5. Add zucchini noodles, cherry tomatoes, basil, and lemon juice. Toss to coat.
6. Simmer for 2-3 minutes, or until zucchini noodles are somewhat softened.
7. Season with salt and pepper to taste.
8. Serve with a sprinkling of Parmesan cheese, if preferred.

Nutritional Information: (approximate per serving)

Calories: 300-350 | Fat: 10-15g | Carbohydrates: 20-25g | Protein: 30-35g

Spiced Chickpea and Sweet Potato Curry with Coconut Milk:

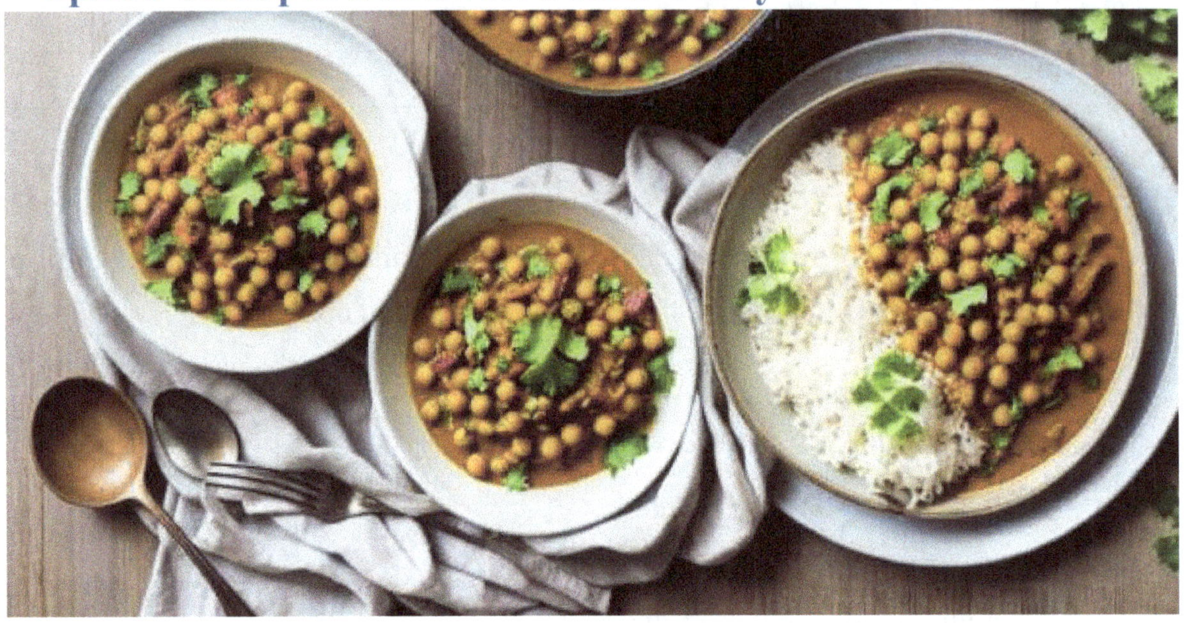

Prep Time: 15 minutes	
Cooking Time: 30-35 minutes	
Total Time: 45-50 minutes	
Serving: 4-6 persons	

Ingredients:

- 2 teaspoons olive oil
- 1 onion, chopped
- 2 cloves garlic, minced
- 1 tablespoon garam masala
- 1 teaspoon turmeric
- 1 teaspoon ginger powder
- 1/2 teaspoon salt
- 1/4 teaspoon black pepper
- 1 big sweet potato, cut into bite-sized pieces
- 1 (15 ounce) can chickpeas, drained and rinsed
- 1 (14 oz) can coconut milk
- Cilantro leaves, for garnish
- Lime wedges, for serving

Directions:

1. Put olive oil in a big pot and heat it on the stove on medium heat.
2. Add onion and simmer for 5 minutes, until softened.
3. Add garlic, garam masala, turmeric, ginger, salt, and pepper. Cook for 1 minute, until aromatic.
4. Stir in sweet potato and chickpeas. Cook for 5 minutes, stirring periodically.
5. Add the coconut milk and heat it up until it starts to gently bubble.
6. Cover and simmer for 20-25 minutes, or until sweet potatoes are cooked.
7. Garnish with cilantro and serve with lime wedges.

Nutritional Information: (approximate per serving)

Calories: 350-400, Fat: 20-25g, Carbohydrates: 40-45g, Protein: 10-15g

Chapter 5: Fish, Shellfish & Chicken Recipes

Seared Scallops with Lemon-Herb Risotto

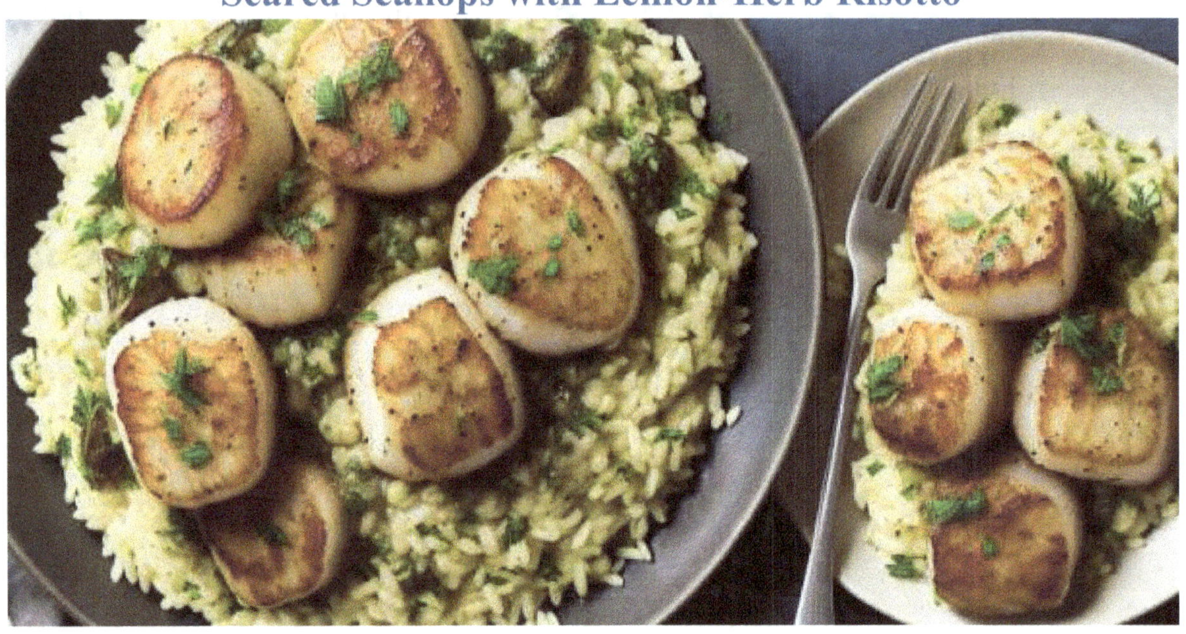

Prep Time: 15 minutes	
Cooking Time: 30-35 minutes	
Total Time: 45-50 minutes	
Serving: 2-3 persons	

Ingredients:

- 12 big sea scallops
- 2 tablespoons olive oil
- Salt and pepper to taste
- 1 cup Arborio rice
- 4 cups chicken broth, warmed
- 1/2 cup dry white wine

- 1 tablespoon lemon zest 1/2 teaspoon dried oregano
- 1/4 teaspoon dried thyme
- 1/4 cup grated Parmesan cheese
- Chopped fresh parsley, for garnish (optional)

Directions:

1. Pat scallops dry and season with salt and pepper.
2. Heat olive oil in a large pan over medium-high heat. Sear scallops for 2-3 minutes each side, until golden brown and caramelized. Transfer to a platter and set aside.
3. In the same skillet, decrease heat to medium and add Arborio rice. Toast for 1 minute, stirring regularly.
4. Add 1/2 cup of heated chicken stock and simmer, stirring regularly, until the rice absorbs the liquid.
5. Gradually add the remaining chicken stock, one ladleful at a time, stirring frequently and allowing the rice to absorb the liquid before adding more. Repeat until the rice is cooked through and creamy, approximately 20-25 minutes.
6. Stir in white wine, lemon zest, oregano, and thyme. Season with salt and pepper to taste.
7. Remove from heat and toss in Parmesan cheese. Add reserved scallops back to the pan and cook through for 1-2 minutes.
8. Garnish with chopped parsley, if preferred.

Nutritional Information: (approximate per serving)

Calories: 500-600 | Fat: 25-30g | Carbohydrates: 50-60g | Protein: 30-35g

Shrimp Saganaki with Feta and Tomatoes:

Prep Time: 10 minutes
Cooking Time: 20-25 minutes
Total Time: 30-35 minutes
Serving: 2-3 persons

Ingredients:

- 1 cup cherry tomatoes, halved
- 1/4 cup Kalamata olives, halved
- 1/2 red onion, finely sliced
- 1/2 pound shrimp, peeled and deveined
- 1/2 cup crumbled feta cheese
- 2 tablespoons olive oil
- 1 teaspoon dried oregano
- 1/4 cup dry white wine (optional)
- 1 tablespoon ouzo (optional)

Directions:

1. Preheat oven to 400°F (200°C).
2. Layer tomatoes, olives, and red onion in a baking dish.
3. Top with shrimp and top with crumbled feta cheese.
4. Drizzle with olive oil and oregano. Add white wine and ouzo, if using.
5. Bake for 20-25 minutes, or until shrimp are cooked through and bubbling.
6. Serve with crusty gluten-free bread for dipping.

Nutritional Information: (approximate per serving)

Calories: 400-500 | Fat: 20-25g | Carbohydrates: 25-30g | Protein: 30-35g

Crispy Baked Cod with Sun-Dried Tomato Pesto:

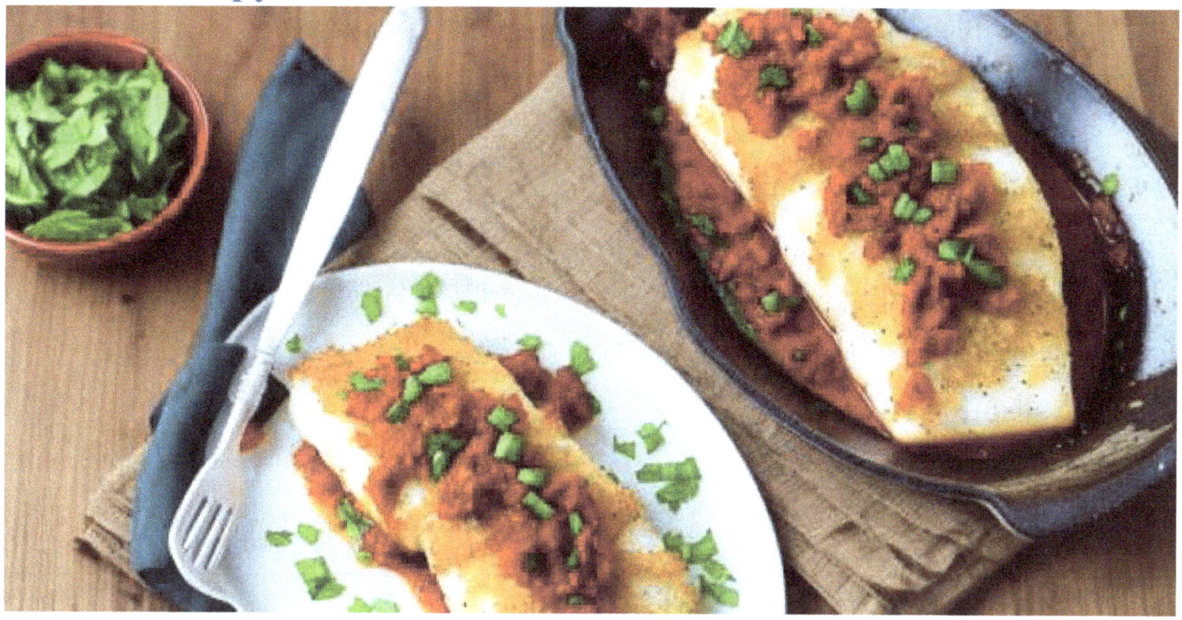

Prep Time: 15 minutes
Cooking Time: 20-25 minutes
Total Time: 35-40 minutes

Ingredients:

- 2 cod fillets
- 1/4 cup sun-dried tomatoes, soaked and chopped
- 1/4 cup pine nuts, roasted
- 1/4 cup fresh basil leaves
- 1/4 cup grated Parmesan cheese
- 1 tablespoon olive oil
- Salt and pepper to taste
- Roasted veggies (zucchini, bell peppers), for serving (optional)

Directions:

1. Preheat oven to 400°F (200°C).
2. In a food processor, blend sun-dried tomatoes, pine nuts, basil, Parmesan cheese, and olive oil. Pulse until a coarse pesto appears.

3. Spread the pesto evenly over the cod fillets.

4. Season with salt and pepper to taste.

5. Place the fish on a baking sheet lined with parchment paper.

6. Bake for 20-25 minutes, or until the fish is flaky and the pesto is slightly crunchy.

7. Serve with roasted veggies, if preferred.

Nutritional Information: (approximate per serving)

Calories: 350-400 | Fat: 20-25g | Carbohydrates: 10-15g | Protein: 30-35g

Mediterranean Chicken Souvlaki Skewers:

Prep Time: 15 minutes plus marinating time
Cooking Time: 15-20 minutes
Total Time: 30-35 minutes + marinating time
Serving: 4-6 persons

Ingredients:

- 1 pound boneless, skinless chicken breasts, cut into pieces
- 1/4 cup olive oil
- Juice of 1 lemon
- 2 cloves garlic, minced
- 1 teaspoon dried oregano
- 1/2 teaspoon paprika
- Salt and pepper to taste
- 1 red bell pepper, cut into pieces
- 1 red onion, cut into wedges
- 1 zucchini, sliced Tzatziki sauce (for serving)

Directions:

1. In a large bowl, add chicken, olive oil, lemon juice, garlic, oregano, paprika, salt, and pepper. Marinate for at least 30 minutes, or up to 4 hours in the refrigerator.

2. Thread chicken, bell peppers, onion, and zucchini onto skewers.

3. Grill or bake skewers over medium heat for 15-20 minutes, or until chicken is cooked through and veggies are soft.

4. Serve with tzatziki sauce.

Nutritional Information: (approximate per serving)

Calories: 300-350 | Fat: 15-20g | Carbohydrates: 10-15g | Protein: 30-35g

Mussels Provençale with Gluten-Free Pasta:

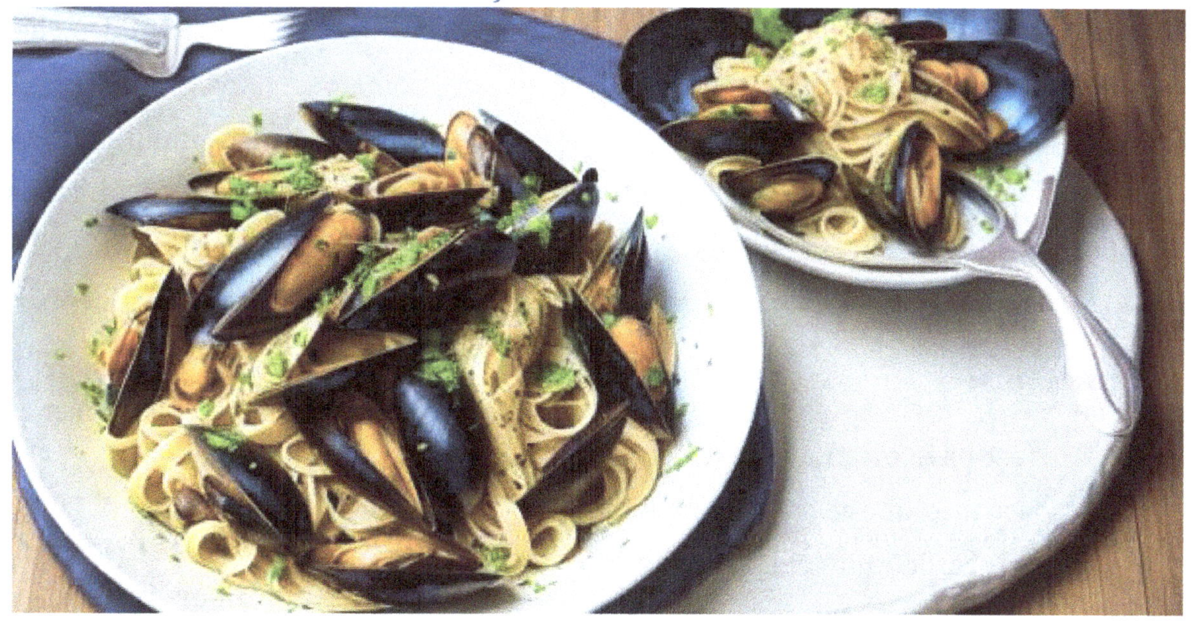

Prep Time: 15 minutes
Cooking Time: 20-25 minutes
Total Time: 35-40 minutes
Serving: 2-3 persons

Ingredients:

- 2 pounds mussels, washed and debearded
- 1/4 cup dry white wine
- 2 shallots, thinly sliced
- 2 cloves garlic, minced
- 1 tablespoon olive oil
- 1/2 teaspoon dried thyme
- 1/4 teaspoon fennel seeds
- 1/4 cup cherry tomatoes, halved
- 1/4 cup chopped fresh parsley
- 1/4 cup gluten-free spaghetti (your favorite kind)
- Salt and pepper to taste
- Parmesan cheese, grated (for serving)

Directions:

1. Heat olive oil in a big saucepan over medium heat. Add shallots and garlic and sauté for 2-3 minutes, until softened.
2. Add thyme, fennel seeds, and white wine. Bring to a simmer.
3. Add mussels and cover the pot. Cook for 5-7 minutes, or until mussels have opened. Discard any mussels that remain unopened.
4. Remove mussels from the saucepan and put aside. Strain the cooking liquid through a fine-mesh strainer into a basin.
5. Cook gluten-free pasta according to package guidelines.
6. In the same saucepan, heat the strained cooking liquid over medium heat. Add cherry tomatoes and parsley and simmer for 2-3 minutes.
7. Add cooked pasta and mussels to the saucepan and stir to coat.
8. Season with salt and pepper to taste.
9. Serve with grated Parmesan cheese.

Nutritional Information: (approximate per serving)

Calories: 400-500 | Fat: 15-20g | Carbohydrates: 40-50g | Protein: 30-35g

Chapter 6: Appetizers & Dips

Whipped Feta with Roasted Grapes and Honey:

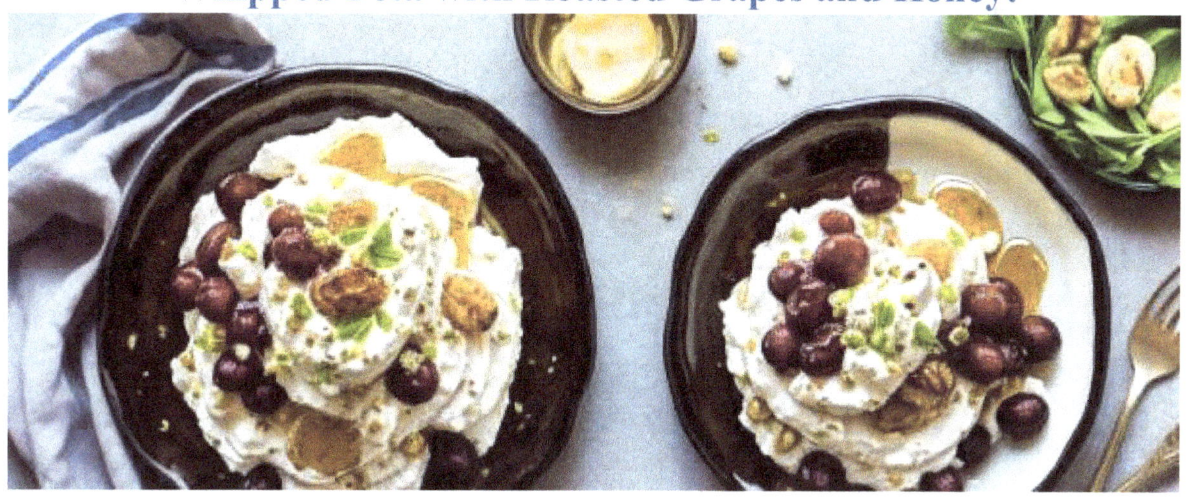

Prep Time: 10 minutes	
Cooking Time: 15-20 minutes (for grapes)	
Total Time: 25-30 minutes	
Serving: 4-6 persons	

Ingredients:

- 8 oz cream cheese, softened
- 4 ounces feta cheese, crumbled
- 1 tablespoon lemon juice
- 1 clove garlic, minced
- 1 tablespoon olive oil
- Salt and pepper to taste
- 1 cup grapes, halved and seeded
- Honey, for drizzling
- Gluten-free crackers or toast points, for serving

Directions:

1. Preheat oven to 400°F (200°C). Toss grapes with a splash of olive oil and put on a baking sheet. Roast for 15-20 minutes, until somewhat softened and caramelized.

2. In a food processor, blend feta cheese, cream cheese, lemon juice, garlic, olive oil, salt, and pepper. Blend until smooth and creamy.

3. Spread creamed feta on crackers or toast points. Top with roasted grapes and sprinkle with honey.

Nutritional Information: (approximate per serving)

Calories: 200-250, Fat: 10-15g, Carbohydrates: 20-25g, Protein: 10-15g

Marinated Olives with Herbs and Citrus

Prep Time: 10 minutes
Marinating Time: 2-4 hours or overnight
Total Time: 2-4 hours (plus marinating)
Serving: 4-6 persons

Ingredients:

- 1 cup green olives (Kalamata, Castelvetrano, or your favorite)
- 1/4 cup olive oil
- Zest of 1 lemon
- 1/2 orange, sliced
- 1 sprig fresh oregano
- 1 sprig fresh thyme
- Pinch of chili flakes
- Crudités like cucumbers, bell peppers, carrots, and celery, for dipping

Directions:

1. In a bowl, add olives, olive oil, lemon zest, orange slices, oregano, thyme, and chili flakes. Toss to coat.

2. Cover and chill for at least 2 hours or overnight for deeper flavor.

3. Serve with different crudités for dipping.

Nutritional Information: (approximate per serving)

Calories: 150-200 | Fat: 15-20g | Carbohydrates: 5-10g | Protein: 1-2g

Pistachio Pesto Stuffed Mini Peppers:

Prep Time: 15 minutes
Cooking Time: 20-25 minutes
Total Time: 35-40 minutes
Serving: 2-3 persons

Ingredients:

- 1/2 cup shelled pistachios
- 1/4 cup fresh basil leaves
- 1 clove garlic, minced
- 1/4 cup olive oil
- Salt and pepper to taste
- 2 baby bell peppers, halved and seeded
- 1/4 cup crumbled feta cheese

Directions:

1. Preheat oven to 400°F (200°C).
2. In a food processor, pulse pistachios until finely chopped. Add basil, garlic, olive oil, salt, and pepper. Blend till a pesto develops.
3. Stuff each pepper half with pesto and top with crumbled feta cheese.
4. Place on a baking pan and bake for 20-25 minutes, until peppers are slightly cooked and feta is golden brown.
5. Serve heated or at room temperature.

Nutritional Information: (approximate per serving)

Calories: 250-300 | Fat: 15-20g | Carbohydrates: 15-20g | Protein: 10-15g

Spicy Chickpea Fritters with Tahini Sauce

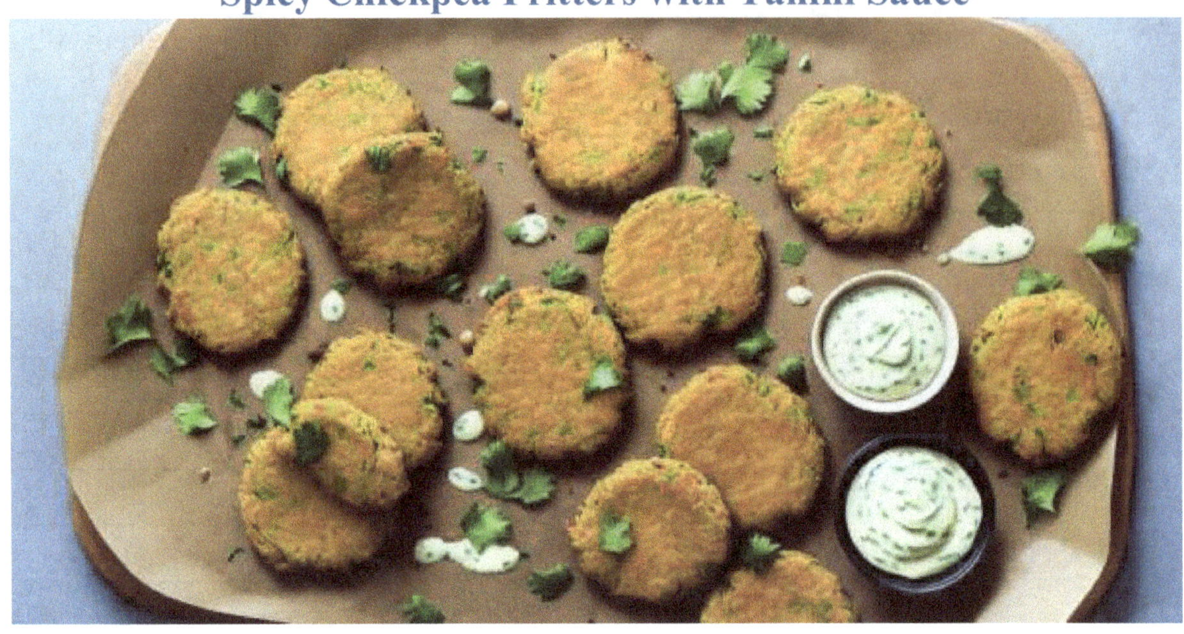

Prep Time: 20 minutes	
Cooking Time: 10-15 minutes	
Total Time: 30-35 minutes	
Serving: 4-6 persons	

Ingredients:

- 1 can (15 oz) chickpeas, drained and rinsed
- 1/4 cup chopped onion
- 1/4 cup chopped fresh parsley
- 1 teaspoon ground cumin
- 1/4 teaspoon cayenne pepper
- Salt and pepper to taste
- Olive oil, for frying 1/4 cup tahini
- 2 teaspoons lemon juice
- 1 clove garlic, minced
- Water, to thin (optional)

Directions:

1. In a large bowl, mash chickpeas using a fork or potato masher until somewhat chunky.

2. Add onion, parsley, cumin, cayenne pepper, salt, and pepper. Mix thoroughly.

3. Form the mixture into tiny patties, approximately 2 inches in diameter.

4. Heat olive oil in a large pan over medium heat.

5. Add the fritters and fry for 3-4 minutes each side, or until golden brown and crispy.

6. To prepare the tahini sauce, whisk together tahini, lemon juice, garlic, and water (if required) to thin the sauce.

7. Serve fritters warm with tahini sauce for dipping.

Nutritional Information: (approximate per serving)

Calories: 250-300 | Fat: 15-20g | Carbohydrates: 20-25g | Protein: 10-15g

Baked Halloumi Bites with Honey and Pomegranate:

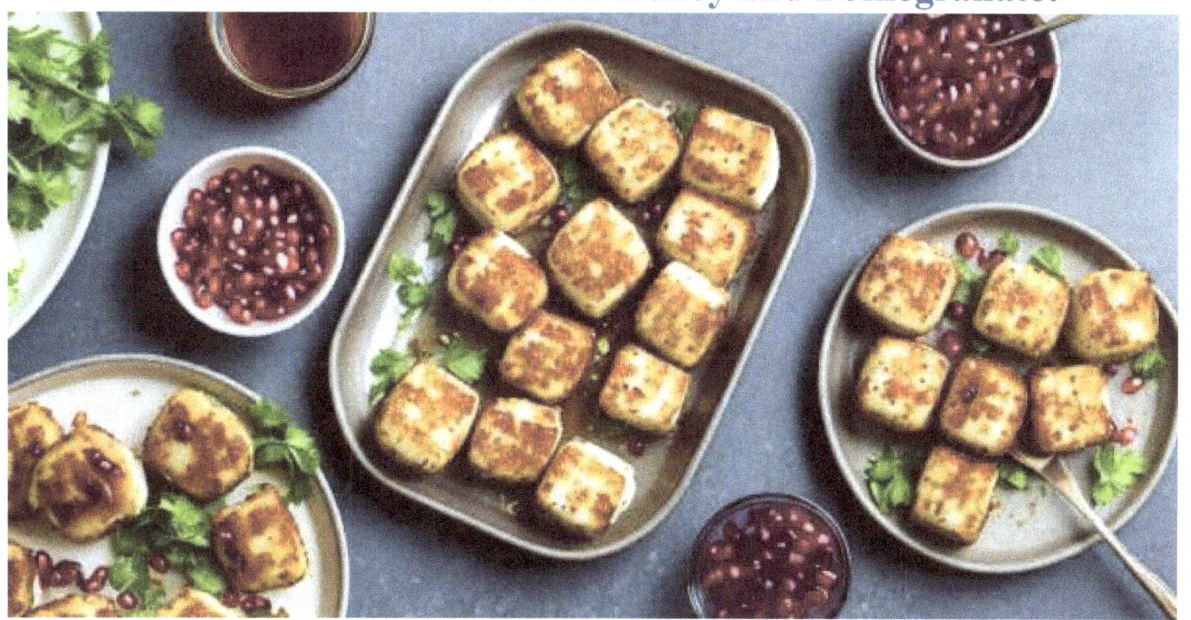

Prep Time: 10 minutes
Cooking Time: 15-20 minutes
Total Time: 25-30 minutes
Serving: 4-6 persons

Ingredients:

- 8 ounces halloumi cheese, chopped into cubes
- 1 tablespoon olive oil
- 1 teaspoon dried oregano
- Pinch of paprika
- Honey, for drizzling
- 1/4 cup pomegranate seeds

Directions:

1. Preheat oven to 400°F (200°C).
2. In a bowl, mix halloumi cubes with olive oil, oregano, and paprika.
3. Spread the cubes on a baking sheet and bake for 15-20 minutes, or until golden brown and somewhat crunchy.
4. Drizzle with honey and sprinkle with pomegranate seeds.
5. Serve heated or at room temperature.

Nutritional Information: (approximate per serving)

Calories: 200-250 | Fat: 15-20g | Carbohydrates: 10-15g | Protein: 10-15g

Chapter 7: Main Courses to Impress: Poultry, Seafood, Vegan & More

Sumac-Crusted Chicken with Lemon-Tahini Sauce and Herb Salad

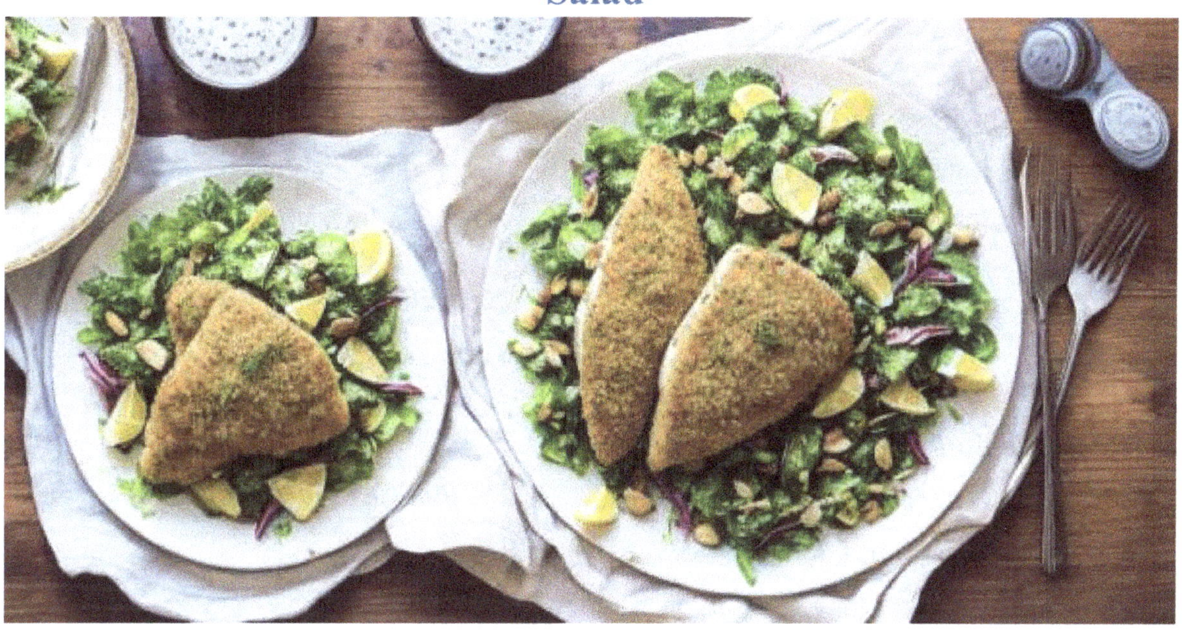

Prep Time: 20 minutes	
Cooking Time: 25-30 minutes	
Total Time: 45-50 minutes	
Serving: 4 persons	

Ingredients:

- 4 boneless, skinless chicken breasts
- 1 tablespoon sumac 1 teaspoon paprika
- 1/2 teaspoon garlic powder
- 1/4 teaspoon salt and pepper
- 2 tablespoons olive oil
- 1/4 cup tahini
- 2 teaspoons lemon juice

- 1/4 cup chopped fresh parsley
- 1 cucumber, chopped
- 1 tomato, chopped
- 1/2 red onion, thinly sliced
- 1/4 cup chopped mint

Directions:

1. Preheat oven to 400°F (200°C).
2. Combine sumac, paprika, garlic powder, salt, and pepper in a bowl. Coat chicken breasts with the spice mixture.
3. Heat olive oil in a large pan over medium-high heat. Sear chicken breasts for 3-4 minutes each side, until golden brown.
4. Transfer chicken to a baking tray and bake for 15-20 minutes, or until cooked through.
5. While chicken cooks, stir together tahini, lemon juice, and parsley in a bowl.
6. Assemble salad with cucumber, tomato, red onion, and mint.
7. Serve chicken with tahini sauce on the side and salad alongside.

Nutritional Information: (approximate per serving)

Calories: 450-500 | Fat: 20-25g | Carbohydrates: 25-30g

| Protein: 40-45g

Roasted Branzino with Fennel and Orange:

Prep Time: 15 minutes
Cooking Time: 25-30 minutes
Total Time: 40-45 minutes
Serving: 4 persons

Ingredients:

- 4 whole branzino fish, cleaned and gutted
- 2 tablespoons olive oil
- Zest of 1 lemon
- 1 sprig fresh thyme

- 1 sprig fresh rosemary
- 1 fennel bulb, thinly sliced
- 1 orange, cut into wedges
- Salt and pepper to taste
- Fingerling potatoes, roasted with garlic and herb oil (optional)

Directions:

1. Preheat oven to 400°F (200°C).
2. Rub olive oil over branzino and season with salt, pepper, lemon zest, thyme, and rosemary. Stuff each fish with fennel and orange wedges.
3. Place fish on a baking pan and roast for 25-30 minutes, or until cooked through and flaky.
4. Serve with roasted fingerling potatoes (optional).

Nutritional Information: (approximate per serving)

Calories: 400-450 | Fat: 15-20g | Carbohydrates: 10-15g | Protein: 40-45g

Crispy Chickpea and Quinoa Stuffed Butternut Squash:

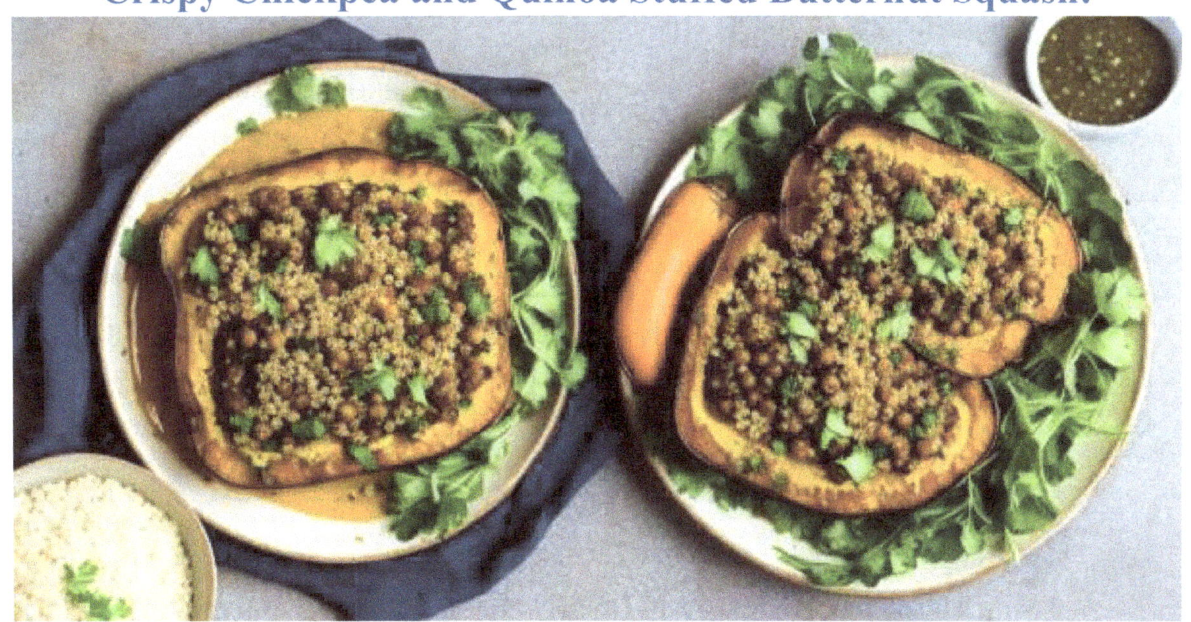

Prep Time: 30 minutes
Cooking Time: 1 hour
Total Time: 1 hour 30 minutes
Serving: 4-6 persons

Ingredients:

- 1 big butternut squash, halved and seeded
- 1 tablespoon olive oil
- Salt and pepper to taste
- 1 cup cooked chickpeas
- 1 cup cooked quinoa
- 1/2 cup sun-dried tomatoes, chopped
- 1 cup spinach, chopped
- 1/2 teaspoon cumin
- 1/4 teaspoon turmeric
- 1/4 cup crumbled feta cheese

Directions:

1. Preheat oven to 400°F (200°C). Brush butternut squash halves with olive oil and season with salt and pepper. Roast for 45-50 minutes, or until tender.
2. While squash roasts, heat olive oil in a pan over medium heat. Add chickpeas, quinoa, sun-dried tomatoes, spinach, cumin, and turmeric. Sauté for 5-7 minutes, until cooked through.
3. Fill roasted squash halves with the chickpea mixture and sprinkle with feta cheese.
4. Bake for 15-20 minutes, or until feta is slightly browned and bubbling.

Nutritional Information: (approximate per serving)

Calories: 500-550 | Fat: 20-25g | Carbohydrates: 60-65g | Protein: 20-25g

Grilled Octopus with Lemony White Bean Salad:

Prep Time: 45 minutes (including tenderizing octopus)
Cooking Time: 20-25 minutes
Total Time: 1 hour 5 minutes
Serving: 4 persons

Ingredients:

- 1-pound octopus legs, washed and tenderized
- 2 tablespoons olive oil
- Salt and pepper to taste
- 1 can (15 oz) white beans, washed and drained
- 1 cucumber, chopped
- 1 tomato, chopped
- 1/2 red onion, thinly sliced
- 1/4 cup chopped fresh parsley
- 2 teaspoons lemon juice
- 1 tablespoon olive oil
- 1/4 teaspoon dried oregano
- 1/4 cup Kalamata olives, chopped

Directions:

1. Tenderize octopus legs using your chosen technique (this commonly includes freezing and thawing, boiling, or using a pressure cooker).
2. Heat olive oil in a grill pan or skillet over medium-high heat. Grill octopus legs for 3-4 minutes each side, until blackened and slightly crispy.
3. In a bowl, add white beans, cucumber, tomato, red onion, parsley, lemon juice, olive oil, oregano, and salt and pepper to taste.
4. Serve grilled octopus on a bed of white bean salad. Top with Kalamata olives.

Nutritional Information: (approximate per serving)

Calories: 400-450 | Fat: 20-25g | Carbohydrates: 30-35g | Protein: 30-35g

Lentil and Artichoke Moussaka with Almond Bechamel

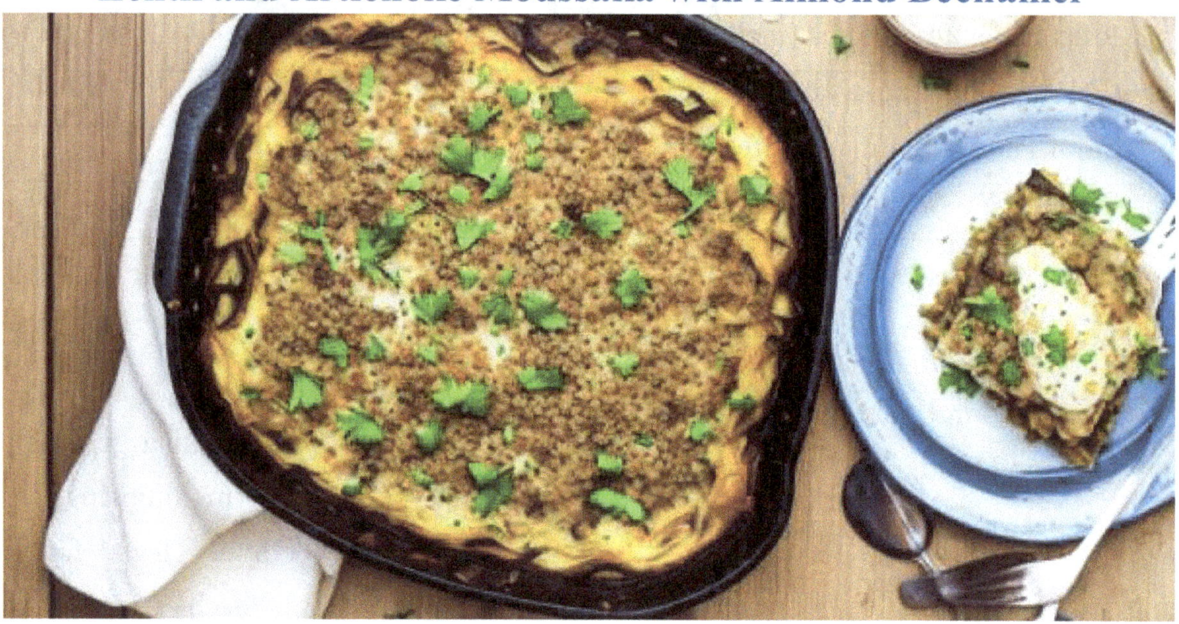

Prep Time: 45 minutes	
Cooking Time: 1 hour	
Total Time: 1 hour 45 minutes	
Serving: 6-8 persons	

Ingredients:

- 1 big eggplant, cut into
- 1/2-inch rounds
- Olive oil, for brushing
- Salt and pepper to taste
- 1 tablespoon olive oil
- 1 onion, chopped 2 cloves garlic, minced
- 1 cup dry lentils, cooked

- 1 can (14 oz) artichoke hearts, drained and diced
- 1/2 teaspoon dried oregano
- 1/4 teaspoon ground cumin
- 1/4 cup chopped fresh parsley
- For the almond bechamel:
- 1/4 cup almond flour
- 2 tablespoons olive oil
- 2 cups vegetable broth

- 1/4 teaspoon salt
- 1/4 teaspoon nutmeg

Directions:

1. Preheat oven to 400°F (200°C). Brush eggplant slices with olive oil and season with salt and pepper. Roast for 20-25 minutes, or until tender.
2. While eggplant roasts, heat olive oil in a pan over medium heat. Add onion and garlic, and simmer for 5 minutes, until softened.
3. Stir in lentils, artichoke hearts, oregano, cumin, and parsley. Cook for 5-7 minutes, until heated through.
4. To create the almond bechamel, mix together almond flour and olive oil in a skillet over medium heat. Gradually stir in veggie broth until smooth.
5. Bring to a boil and cook for 5-7 minutes, until thickened. Stir in salt and nutmeg.
6. In a baking dish, place half of the eggplant slices, followed by the lentil mixture, and then the remaining eggplant pieces.
7. Pour the almond bechamel over the top and bake for 30-35 minutes, or until golden brown and bubbling.
8. Let cool slightly before serving.

Nutritional Information: (approximate per serving)

Calories: 350-400 | Fat: 15-20g | Carbohydrates: 40-45g | Protein: 20-25g

Chapter 8: Soup Recipes

Lentil Soup:

Prep Time: 10 minutes
Cooking Time: 45 minutes
Total Time: 55 minutes
Servings: 6

Ingredients:

- 2 cups of lentils, washed and drained
- 1 onion, chopped
- 2 carrots, chopped
- 2 celery stalks, chopped
- 4 garlic cloves, minced
- 1 teaspoon of cumin
- 1 teaspoon of coriander
- 1 teaspoon of turmeric
- 6 cups of vegetable broth
- Salt and pepper to taste

Directions:

1. In a big saucepan, heat some oil over medium heat.
2. Add the onion, carrots, and celery, and simmer until the veggies are soft.
3. Add the garlic, cumin, coriander, and turmeric, and simmer for another minute.
4. Add the lentils and vegetable broth, and bring to a boil.
5. Reduce the heat and simmer for 30-40 minutes, or until the lentils are cooked.
6. Season with salt and pepper to taste.

Nutritional Value:

Each serving of this soup includes around 200 calories, 13g of protein, and 10g of fiber.

Avgolemono Soup:

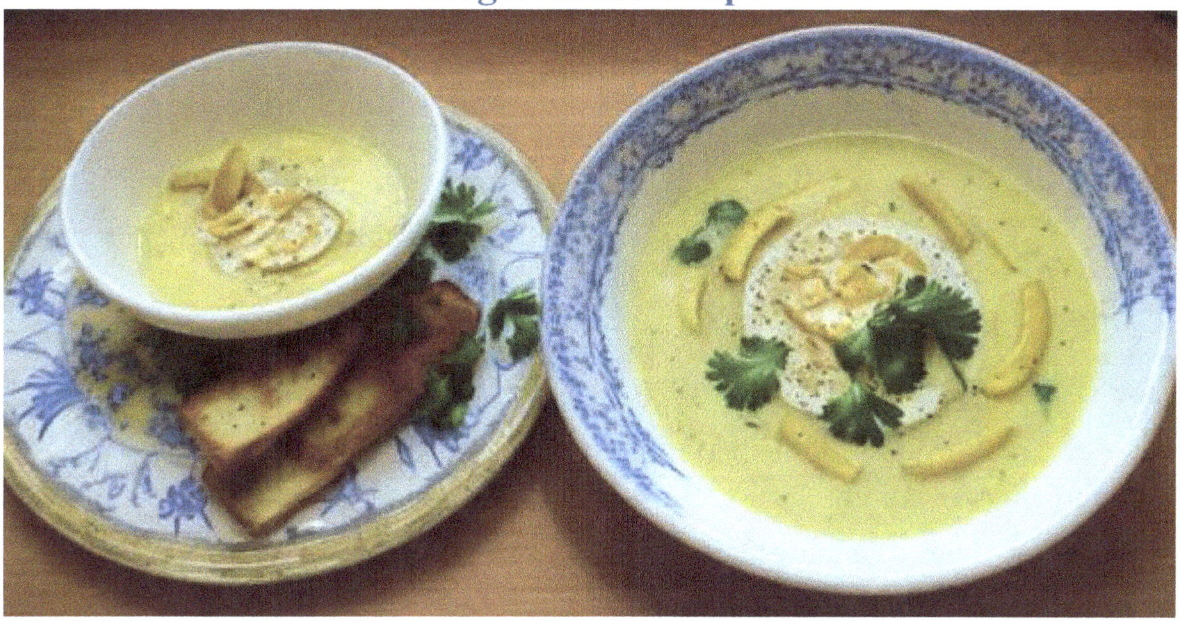

Prep Time: 10 minutes
Cooking Time: 30 minutes
Total Time: 40 minutes
Servings: 4

Ingredients:

- 4 cups of chicken broth
- 1/2 cup of rice
- 2 eggs
- 1/4 cup of lemon juice
- Salt and pepper to taste

Directions:

1. In a big pot, heat up the chicken broth until it starts to bubble and steam..
2. Add the rice, decrease the heat, and simmer for 20-25 minutes, or until the rice is cooked.
3. In a small bowl, mix together the eggs and lemon juice.

4. Slowly add 1 cup of the heated broth to the egg mixture, whisking continuously.

5. Pour the egg mixture back into the saucepan, and stir until the soup is thickened.

6. Season with salt and pepper to taste.

Nutritional Value:

Each serving of this soup includes around 150 calories, 8g of protein, and 1g of fiber.

Chickpea and Vegetable Soup:

Prep Time: 15 minutes
Cooking Time: 30 minutes
Total Time: 45 minutes
Servings: 4

Ingredients:

- 1 tablespoon of olive oil
- 1 onion, chopped 2 garlic cloves, minced
- 1 red bell pepper, chopped
- 1 zucchini, chopped
- 1 can of chickpeas, washed and drained
- 4 cups of vegetable broth
- 1/4 cup of fresh lime juice
- Salt and pepper to taste

Directions:

1. In a big pot, warm up the olive oil on the stove at a medium temperature.

2. Add the onion and garlic, and sauté until the veggies are soft.

3. Add the red bell pepper and zucchini, and simmer for another 5 minutes.

4. Add the chickpeas and vegetable broth, and bring to a boil.

5. Lower the heat and let it cook gently for 15-20 minutes, until the vegetables are easy to bite.

6. Mix in the lime juice and add some salt and pepper to make it taste good.

Nutritional Value:

Each serving of this soup includes around 200 calories, 8g of protein, and 8g of fiber

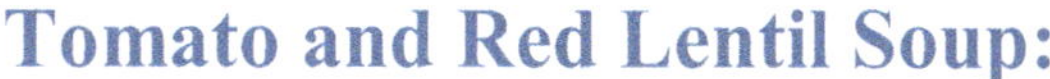

Tomato and Red Lentil Soup:

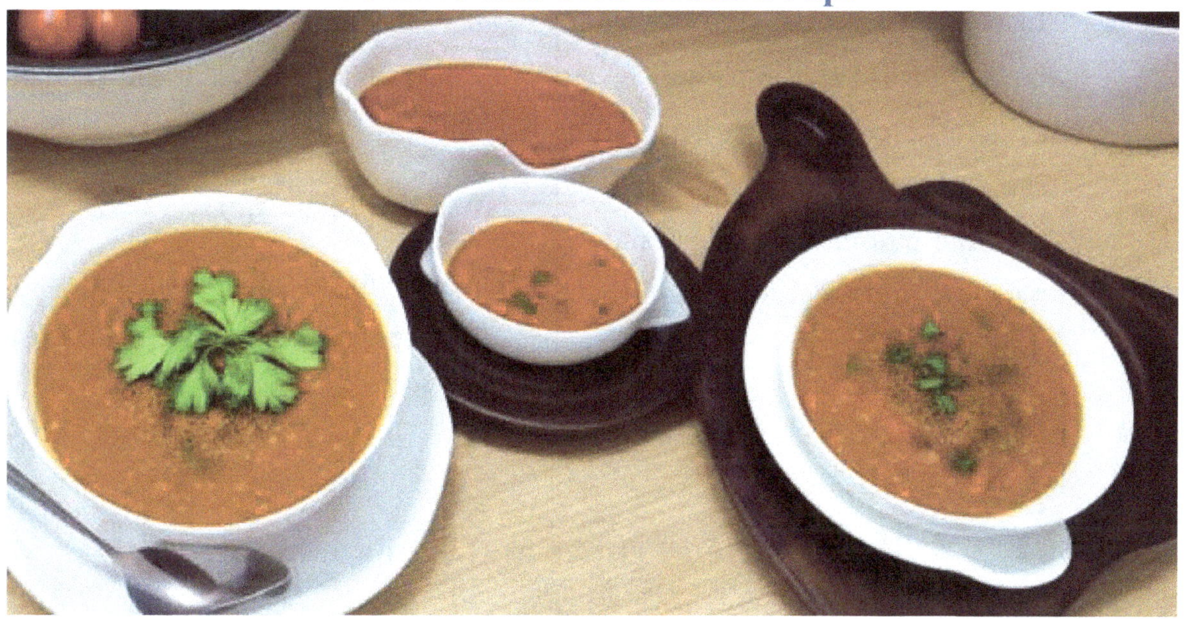

Prep Time: 10 minutes
Cooking Time: 30 minutes
Total Time: 40 minutes
Servings: 4

Ingredients:

- 1 tablespoon of olive oil
- 1 onion, chopped

- 2 garlic cloves, minced
- 1 teaspoon of cumin
- 1 teaspoon of coriander
- 1/2 teaspoon of paprika

- 1 can of chopped tomatoes
- 1 cup of red lentils, washed and drained
- 4 cups of vegetable broth
- Salt and pepper to taste

Directions:

1. In a big pot, warm up the olive oil on the stove at medium heat.
2. Add the onion and garlic, and sauté until the veggies are soft.
3. Add the cumin, coriander, and paprika, and heat for another minute.
4. Put the chopped tomatoes, red lentils, and vegetable broth in a pot and heat it up until it starts to bubble.
5. Then, turn down the heat and let it cook gently for about 20 to 25 minutes, or until the lentils are soft and ready to eat.
6. Season with salt and pepper to taste.

Nutritional Value:

Each serving of this soup includes about 200 calories, 13g of protein, and 10g of fiber.

Roasted Red Pepper and Tomato Soup:

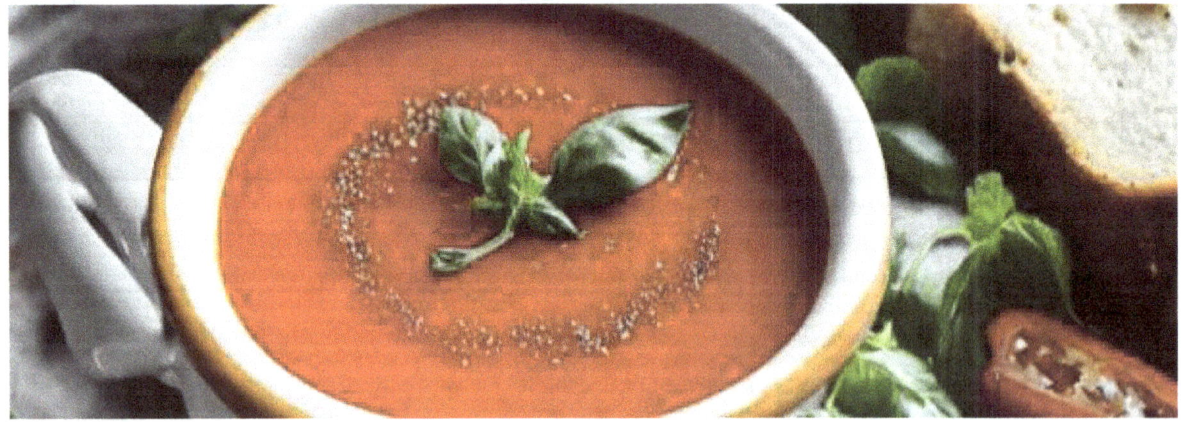

| Prep Time: 10 minutes |
| Cooking Time: 50 minutes |

<table><tr><td>Total Time: 60 minutes</td></tr><tr><td>Servings: 4</td></tr></table>

Ingredients:

- 2 red bell peppers, halved and seeded
- 2 teaspoons of olive oil
- 1 onion, chopped
- 2 garlic cloves, minced
- 1 teaspoon of dried basil
- 1 teaspoon of dried oregano
- 1/2 teaspoon of paprika
- 1 can of chopped tomatoes
- 2 cups of vegetable broth
- Salt and pepper to taste

Directions:

1. Preheat the oven to 400°F.
2. Place the red bell peppers on a baking sheet, cut side down, and roast for 20-25 minutes, or until the skin is roasted and blistered.
3. Remove the peppers from the oven and set them in a basin. Cover the bowl with plastic wrap and let the peppers steam for 10 minutes.
4. Peel the peel off the peppers and slice them into tiny pieces.
5. In a big pot, warm up the olive oil on the stove at medium heat.
6. Add the onion and garlic, and sauté until the veggies are soft.
7. Add the basil, oregano, and paprika, and simmer for another minute.
8. Add the diced tomatoes, roasted red peppers, and vegetable broth, and bring to a boil.
9. Reduce down the heat and let it cook gently for 20-25 minutes, or until the vegetables are nice and soft.
10. Season with salt and pepper to taste.

Nutritional Value:

Each serving of this soup includes about 120 calories, 3g of protein, and 4g of fiber.

Honey-Walnut Baklava Bites:

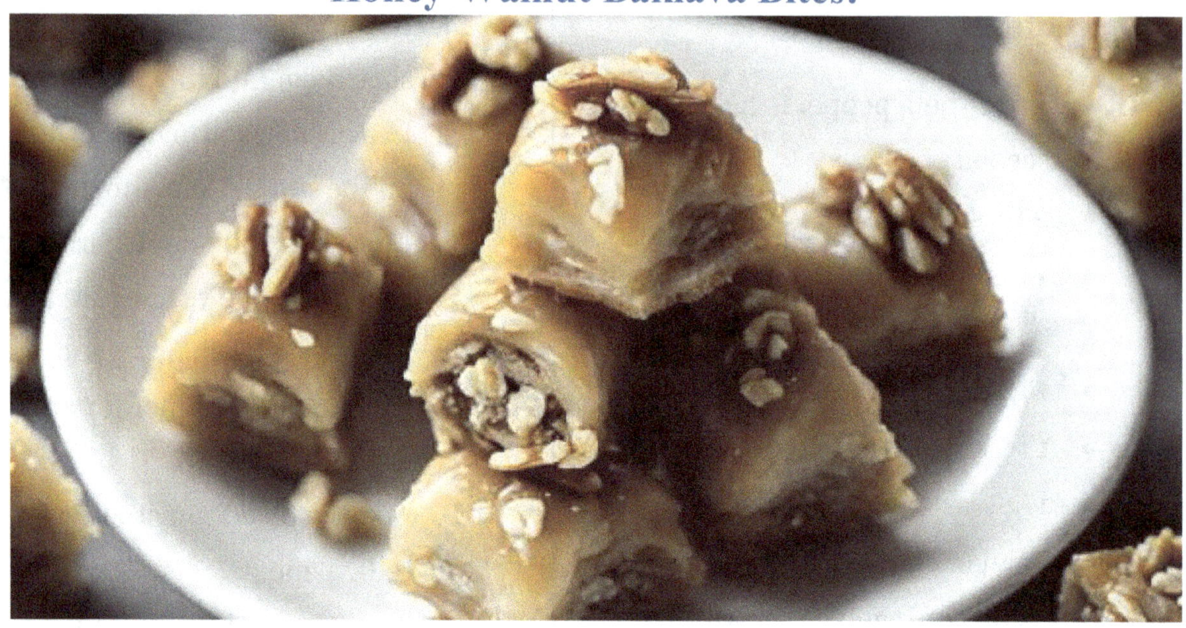

Prep Time: 15 minutes	
Cooking Time: None	
Total Time: 15 minutes	
Serving: 20-25 bites	

Ingredients:

- 1 cup almonds
- 1 cup walnuts
- 1 cup pitted dates
- 1/4 cup honey
- 1/4 cup chopped walnuts, toasted (optional)

Directions:

1. Pulse almonds, walnuts, and dates in a food processor until finely chopped and sticky.
2. Form the mixture into little squares or balls.

3. Drizzle with honey and sprinkle with toasted walnuts, if preferred.

4. Put it in the refrigerator and wait for 30 minutes before you can eat it.

Nutritional Information: (approximate per serving)

Calories: 100-125 | Fat: 5-7g | Carbohydrates: 15-20g | Protein: 2-3g

Greek Yogurt Panna Cotta with Berries and Pistachios

Prep Time: 10 minutes
Setting Time: 4 hours Total Time: 4 hours 10 minutes
Serving: 4-6 tiny servings

Ingredients:

- 1 cup plain Greek yogurt
- 1/2 cup honey
- 1 teaspoon vanilla extract
- 1 teaspoon unflavored gelatin powder
- 1/4 cup cold water
- 1 cup fresh berries (strawberries, raspberries, blueberries)
- 1/4 cup chopped pistachios

Directions:

1. Put the gelatin in a bowl of cold water and let it sit for 5 minutes.

2. Whisk together yogurt, honey, and vanilla extract.

3. Heat gelatin in a small saucepan over low heat until melted. Stir into yogurt mixture.

4. Divide among tiny serving cups or jars. Refrigerate for at least 4 hours to set.

5. Top with berries and pistachios before serving.

Nutritional Information: (approximate per serving)

Calories: 200-250, Fat: 5-7g, Carbohydrates: 30-35g, Protein: 15-20g

Spiced Almond Flour Cookies with Lemon Glaze

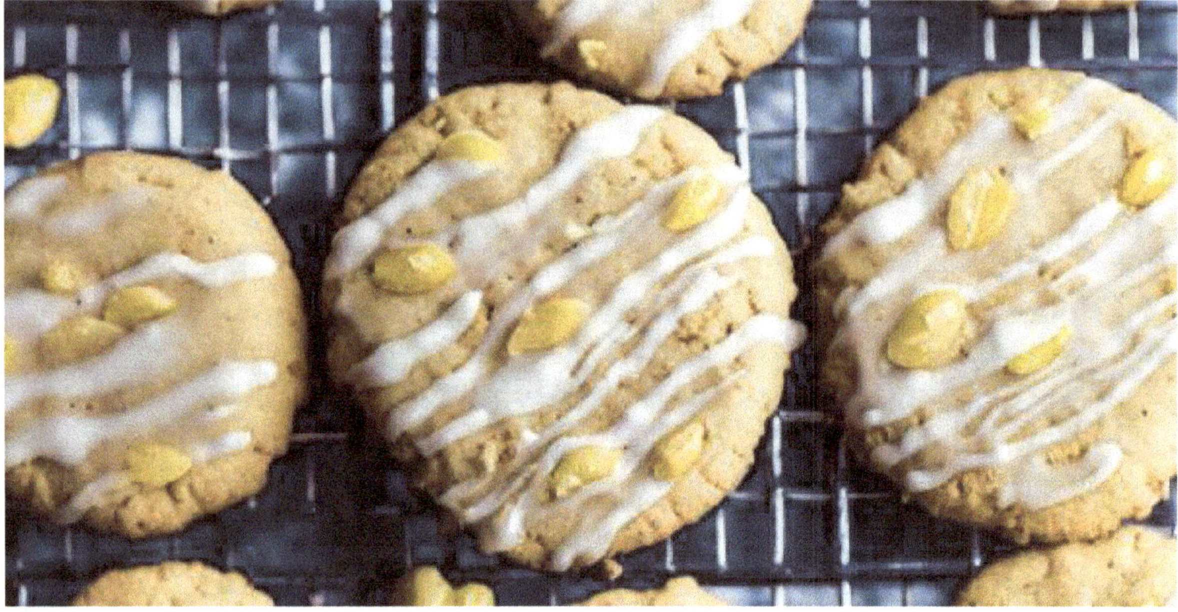

Prep Time: 15 minutes	
Cooking Time: 12-15 minutes	
Total Time: 27-30 minutes	
Serving: 12-15 cookies	

Ingredients:

- 1 cup almond flour
- 1/2 cup coconut sugar
- 1/2 teaspoon baking powder
- 1/4 teaspoon cardamom
- 1/4 teaspoon cinnamon
- 1/4 teaspoon salt
- 1 egg
- 1/4 cup coconut oil, melted
- 1/4 cup powdered sugar
- 1 tablespoon lemon juice
- Pinch of salt

Directions:

1. Preheat oven to 350°F (175°C). Cover a baking sheet with parchment paper in order to prevent the food from sticking to the surface.

2. In a bowl, mix together almond flour, coconut sugar, baking powder, spices, and salt.

3. In a separate dish, mix together egg and melted coconut oil. Mix the dry ingredients together and stir until they become a thick dough. Then, take spoonful of the dough and place them on a baking sheet. Put the baking sheet in the oven and cook for 12-15 minutes, or until the dough turns a nice golden-brown color.

4. To prepare the glaze, mix together powdered sugar, lemon juice, and a bit of salt. Drizzle over cooled cookies.

Nutritional Information: (approximate per cookie)

Calories: 150-175 | Fat: 10-12g | Carbohydrates: 15-20g | Protein: 2-3g

Roasted Figs with Honey and Mascarpone:

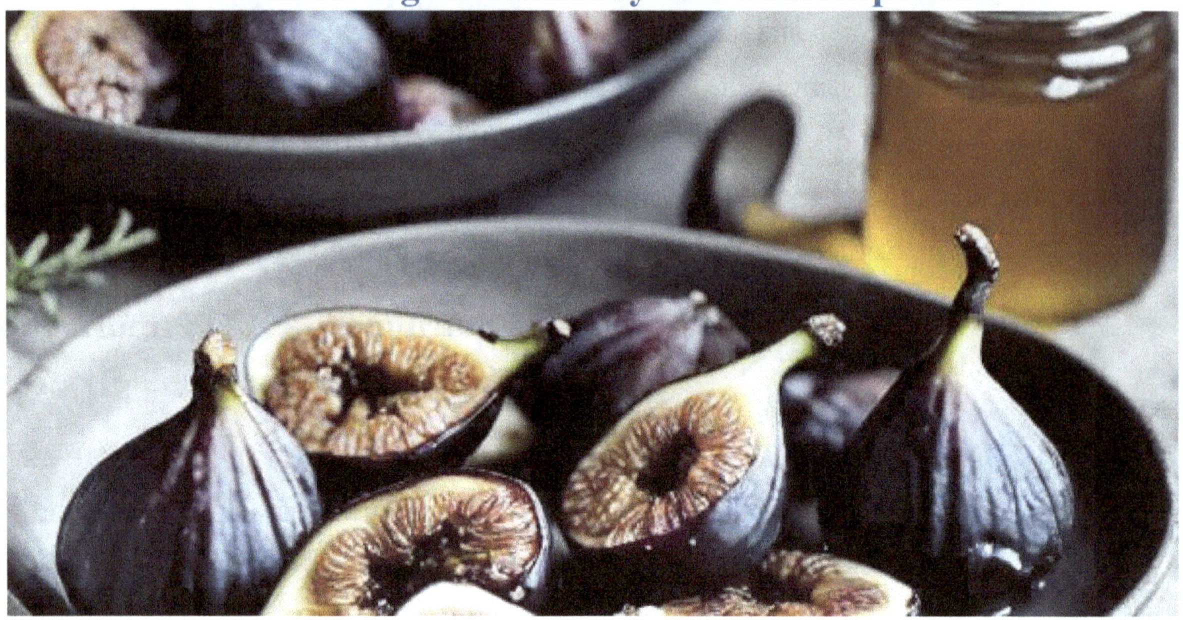

Prep Time: 10 minutes	
Cooking Time: 15-20 minutes	
Total Time: 25-30 minutes	
Serving: 4-6 servings	

Ingredients:

- 4-6 fresh figs, halved
- 2 tablespoons honey
- 1 tablespoon balsamic vinegar
- 1 sprig fresh thyme
- Mascarpone cheese, for serving

Directions:

1. Preheat oven to 400°F (200°C).

2. Arrange fig halves, cut-side up, on a baking sheet. Drizzle with honey and balsamic vinegar. Top each fig with a tiny sprig of thyme.

3. Roast for 15-20 minutes, or until figs are softened and slightly caramelized.

4. Serve warm with dollops of mascarpone cheese.

Nutritional Information:

(approximate per serving)

Calories: 150-200 | Fat: 5-7g | Carbohydrates: 25-30g | Protein: 2-3g

Date and Walnut Stuffed Medjool Dates:

Prep Time: 15 minutes
Cooking Time: None
Total Time: 15 minutes
Serving: 10-12 stuffed dates

Ingredients:

10-12 Medjool dates, pitted

1/2 cup chopped walnuts

1/4 cup chopped almonds

1/2 teaspoon cinnamon

1 tablespoon maple syrup

1/4 cup dark chocolate, melted (optional)

Directions:

Combine walnuts, almonds, cinnamon, and maple syrup in a bowl.

Fill each date with the nut mixture.

Drizzle with melted dark chocolate, if preferred.

Refrigerate for at least 30 minutes to enable flavors to combine.

Nutritional Information: (approximate per serving)

Calories: 150-175 | Fat: 5-7g | Carbohydrates: 25-30g | Protein: 2-3g

Chapter 10: 7-Day Diet Meal Plan

Day 1

Breakfast: Greek yogurt with honey and berries

Prep Time: 5 minutes
Total Time: 5 minutes
Servings: 1

Ingredients:

- 3/4 cup of Greek yogurt
- 1/2 cup of blueberries
- 1 cup of chopped strawberries
- 1 tablespoon of honey

Directions:

1. Place 3/4 cup of Greek yogurt in a bowl.

2. Get your berries and cut them up. Put the pieces on top of the yogurt.
3. Drizzle honey over top.
4. Enjoy as an amazing breakfast!

Nutritional Value:

Each serving of this meal contains approximately 240 calories, 16g of protein, and 44g of carbohydrates.

Lunch: Chickpea and vegetable soup

Prep Time: 10 minutes
Cooking Time: 25 minutes
Total Time: 35 minutes
Servings: 8

Ingredients:

- 2 tablespoons of butter
- 2 tablespoons of olive oil
- 1 onion, chopped
- 2 carrots, chopped
- 2 celery stalks, chopped
- 4 garlic cloves, minced
- 1 bay leaf
- Salt and pepper to taste
- 2 cans of chickpeas, rinsed and drained
- 1 can of diced tomatoes
- 6 cups of vegetable broth
- 1/2 teaspoon of turmeric

Directions:

1. In a soup pot, heat the oil and butter over medium heat.

2. Add the celery, garlic, onions, carrots, bay leaf, salt, and pepper. Cook, stirring often, for 6 to 8 minutes, or until the veggies are soft.

3. Add the tomatoes and chickpeas, and season with turmeric.

4. Once added, bring the vegetable broth to a boil.

5. Reduce heat and simmer for 15-20 minutes.

6. Season with salt and pepper to taste.

Nutritional Value:

Each serving of this meal contains approximately 200 calories, 8g of protein, and 8g of fiber.

Dinner: Grilled salmon with roasted vegetables

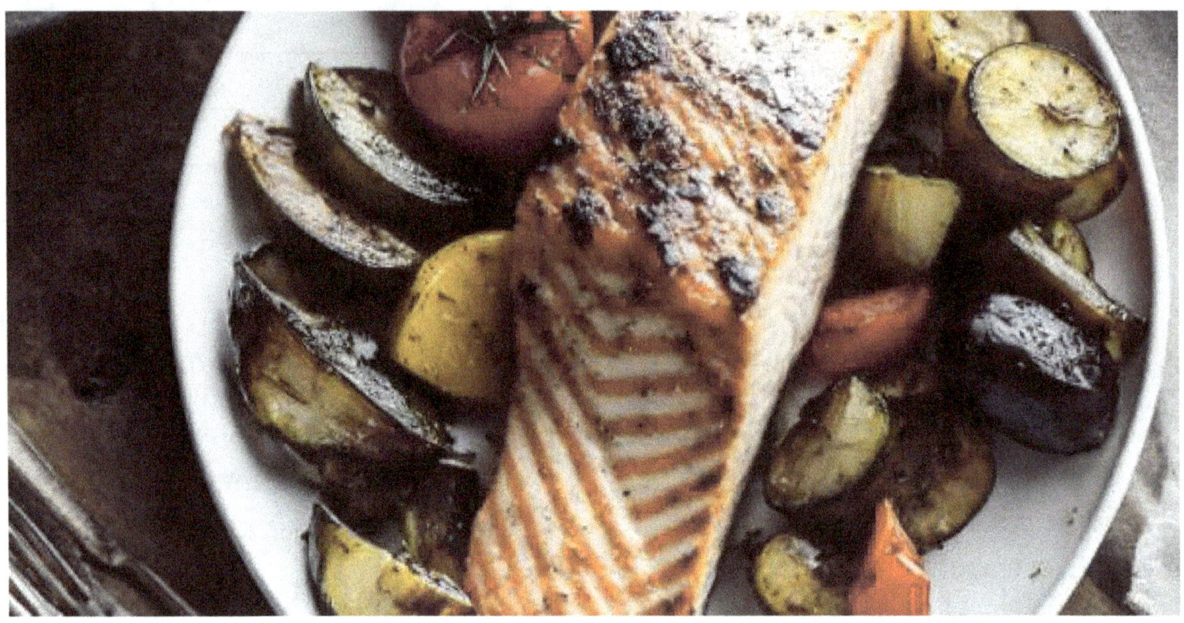

| Prep Time: 25 minutes |
| Cooking Time: 20 minutes |
| Total Time: 45 minutes |
| Servings: 4 |

Ingredients:

1 medium zucchini, halved lengthwise

Two bell peppers, either red, orange, or yellow, cut, split, and seeded

One medium red onion, thinly sliced into 1-inch pieces

1 tablespoon of extra-virgin olive oil

1/2 teaspoon of salt, divided

1/2 teaspoon of ground pepper

1 1/4 pounds of salmon fillet, cut into 4 portions

1/4 cup of thinly sliced fresh basil

1 lemon, cut into 4 wedges

Directions:

1. Preheat grill to medium-high.

2. After applying oil to the zucchini, peppers, and onion, season with 1/4 teaspoon salt.

3. Add pepper and the remaining 1/4 teaspoon of salt to the fish.

4. Arrange the veggies and salmon slices on the grill with the skin side down.

5. Cook the veggies for 4 to 6 minutes on each side, turning them once or twice, or until they are just soft and have grill marks.

6. Fry the salmon for 8 to 10 minutes, or until it flakes when examined with a fork, without flipping it.

7. Once the veggies have cooled down enough, coarsely chop them and combine them in a big dish.

8. If preferred, remove the skin off the salmon fillets and serve with the veggies.

9. Serve each dish with a lemon slice and garnish with one tablespoon of basil.

Nutritional Value:

Each serving of this meal contains approximately 281 calories, 13g of fat, 11g of carbohydrates, and 30g of protein.

Snack: Apple slices with almond butter

Prep Time: 5 minutes
Total Time: 5 minutes
Servings: 1

Ingredients:

- 1 medium apple, sliced
- 3 tablespoons of almond butter
- 2 teaspoons of shredded unsweetened coconut

Directions:

1. Core and slice the apple of your choice.

2. Spoon some almond butter into a bowl.

3. Drizzle almond butter over the apple slices.

4. Sprinkle shredded unsweetened coconut over the almond butter.

5. Enjoy this healthy snack!

Nutritional Value:

Each serving of this snack contains approximately 115 calories, 2g of protein, and 4g of fat

Breakfast: Scrambled eggs mixed with spinach and feta cheese

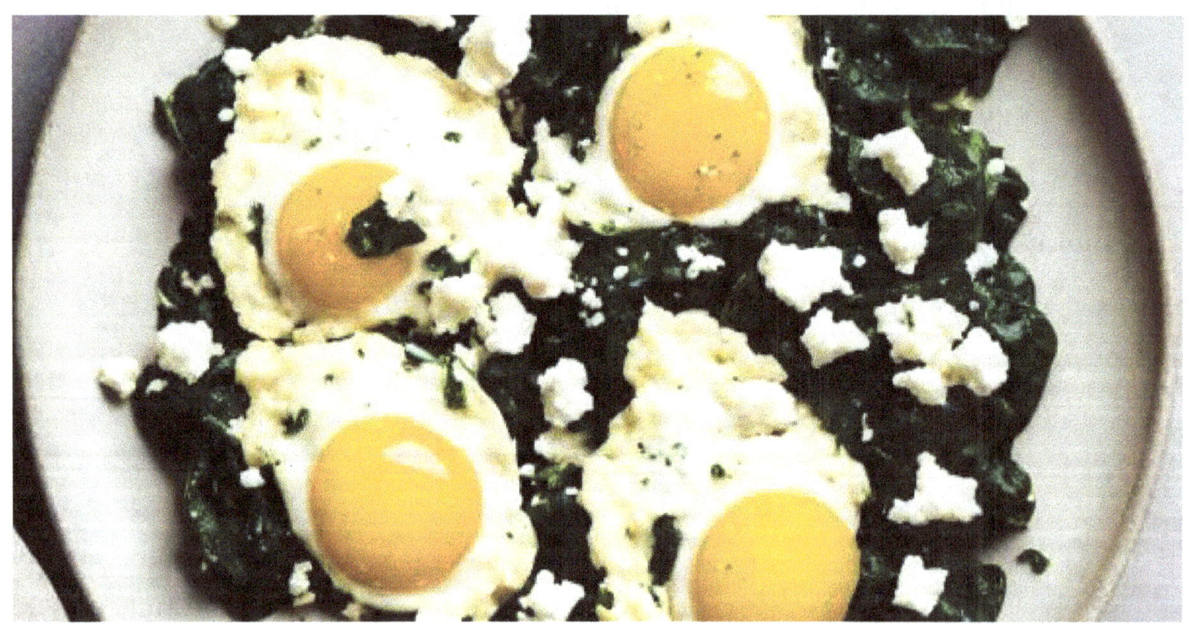

Prep Time: 5 minutes

| Cooking Time: 5 minutes |
| Total Time: 10 minutes |
| Servings: 1 |

Ingredients:

- 3/4 cup of fresh spinach
- 4 large eggs
- 1 tablespoon of butter
- 1 oz. of feta cheese
- 1 pinch of crushed red pepper
- 1 pinch of freshly cracked black pepper
- 1 pinch of salt

Directions:

1. In a big pan, make the butter liquid by heating it on medium heat.
2. Add the spinach and cook until wilted.
3. In a mixing bowl, whisk together the eggs, salt, black pepper, and crushed red pepper.
4. Carefully pour the egg mixture into the pan and cook it until the eggs are fully cooked and not runny anymore.
5. Crumble the feta cheese over the eggs and serve hot.

Nutritional Value:

Each serving of this meal contains approximately 240 calories, 16g of protein, and 44g of carbohydrates.

Lunch: Quinoa salad with grilled chicken

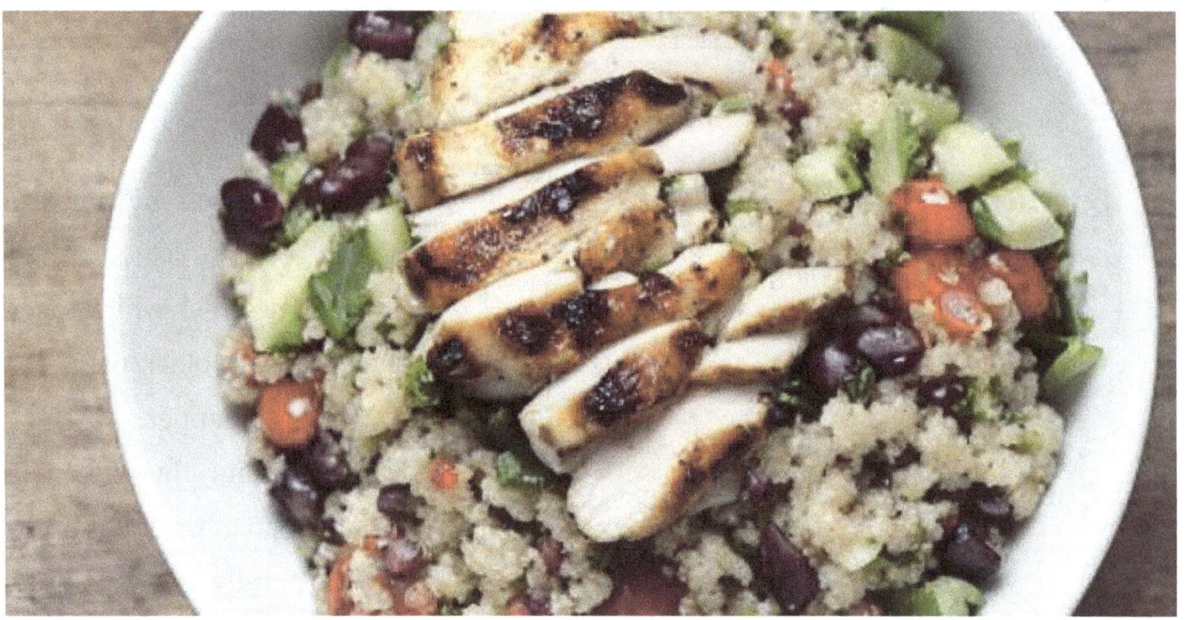

| Prep Time: 10 minutes |
| Cooking Time: 20 minutes |
| Total Time: 30 minutes |
| Servings: 4 |

Ingredients:

- 1 cup of quinoa
- 2 cups of water
- 1/4 cup of olive oil
- 1/4 cup of lemon juice
- 1 teaspoon of honey
- 1/2 teaspoon of salt
- 1/4 teaspoon of black pepper
- 2 cups of cooked chicken, diced
- 1/2 cup of red onion, diced
- 1/2 cup of cucumber, diced
- 1/2 cup of cherry tomatoes, halved
- 1/4 cup of fresh parsley, chopped

Directions:

1. Rinse the quinoa in a fine-mesh strainer and place it in a saucepan with 2 cups of water.
2. Bring the quinoa to a boil, then reduce the heat and simmer for 15-20 minutes, or until the quinoa is tender.
3. In a mixing bowl, whisk together the olive oil, lemon juice, honey, salt, and black pepper.
4. Add the cooked quinoa, chicken, red onion, cucumber, cherry tomatoes, and parsley to the mixing bowl and toss until everything is coated in the dressing.
5. Serve chilled.

Nutritional Value:

Each serving of this meal contains approximately 350 calories, 25g of protein, and 25g of carbohydrates.

Dinner: Baked chicken with roasted sweet potatoes

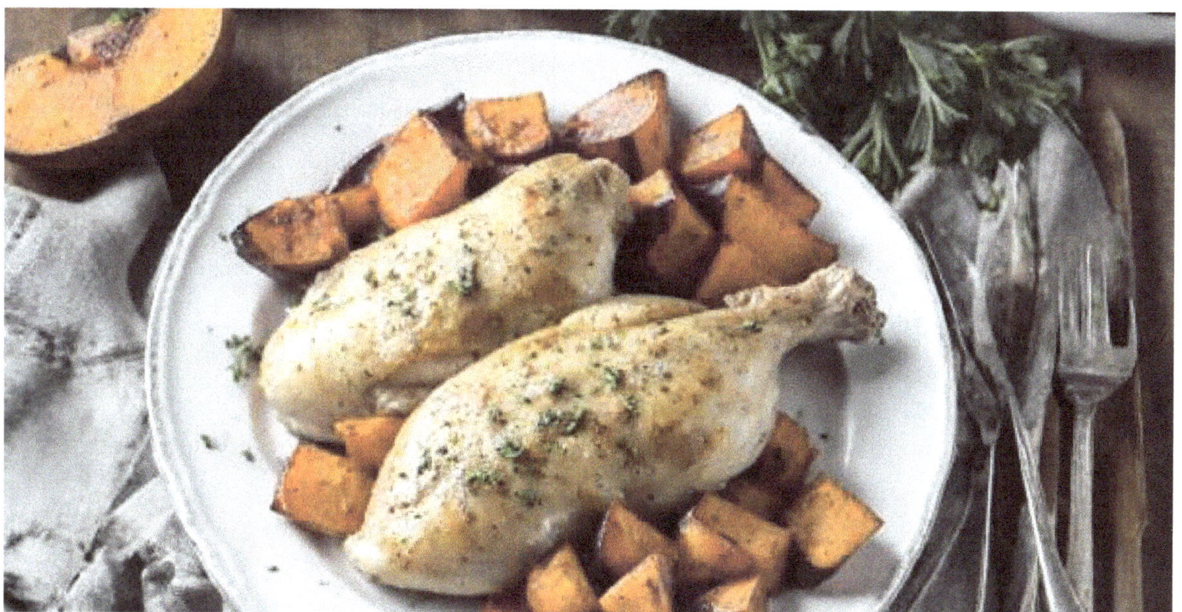

Prep Time: 10 minutes

| Cooking Time: 40 minutes |
| Total Time: 50 minutes |
| Servings: 4 |

Ingredients:

- 4 boneless, skinless chicken breasts
- 2 large sweet potatoes, peeled and cubed
- 2 tablespoons of olive oil
- 1 teaspoon of garlic powder
- 1 teaspoon of paprika
- 1/2 teaspoon of salt
- 1/4 teaspoon of black pepper

Directions:

1. Preheat the oven to 400°F.
2. In a mixing bowl, whisk together the olive oil, garlic powder, paprika, salt, and black pepper.
3. Add the cubed sweet potatoes to the mixing bowl and toss until they are coated in the seasoning.
4. Place the chicken breasts and sweet potatoes on a baking sheet and bake for 35-40 minutes, or until the chicken is cooked through and the sweet potatoes are tender.
5. Serve hot.

Nutritional Value:

Each serving of this meal contains approximately 300 calories, 25g of protein, and 20g of carbohydrates.

Snack: Carrots with hummus

Prep Time: 5 minutes
Total Time: 5 minutes
Servings: 1

Ingredients:

- 1 cup of baby carrots
- 3 tablespoons of hummus

Directions:

1. Arrange the baby carrots on a plate.
2. Spoon the hummus into a small bowl.
3. Dip the carrots into the hummus and enjoy!

Nutritional Value:

Each serving of this snack contains approximately 100 calories, 2g of protein, and 10g

Breakfast: Gluten-free oatmeal with sliced banana and walnuts

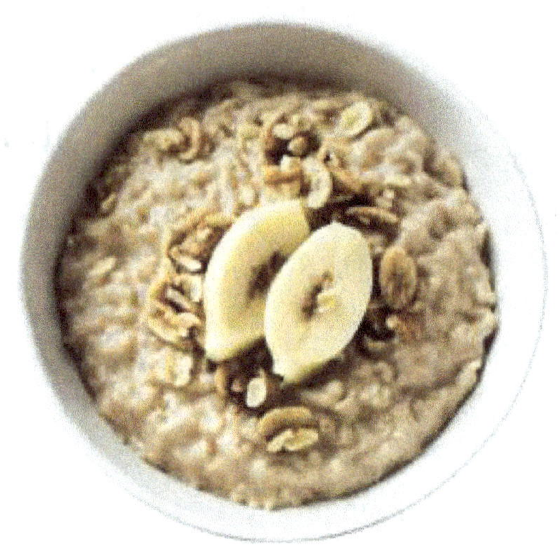

Prep Time: 5 minutes	
Cooking Time: 5 minutes	
Total Time: 10 minutes	
Servings: 1	

Ingredients:

- 1/2 cup of gluten-free quick oats
- 1 cup of water
- 1/2 banana, sliced
- 1 tablespoon of chopped walnuts
- 1 teaspoon of honey

Directions:

1. Put a small pot on the stove and heat up the water until it starts to bubble and get really hot.
2. Add the oats and reduce the heat to low.

3. Cook for 3-5 minutes, stirring occasionally, until the oats are tender and the mixture has thickened.

4. Bring it down from heat and allow it to cool for a minute.

5. Top with sliced banana, chopped walnuts, and honey.

6. Serve hot.

Nutritional Value:

Each serving of this meal contains approximately 250 calories, 6g of protein, and 7g of fiber.

Lunch: Greek salad with grilled shrimp

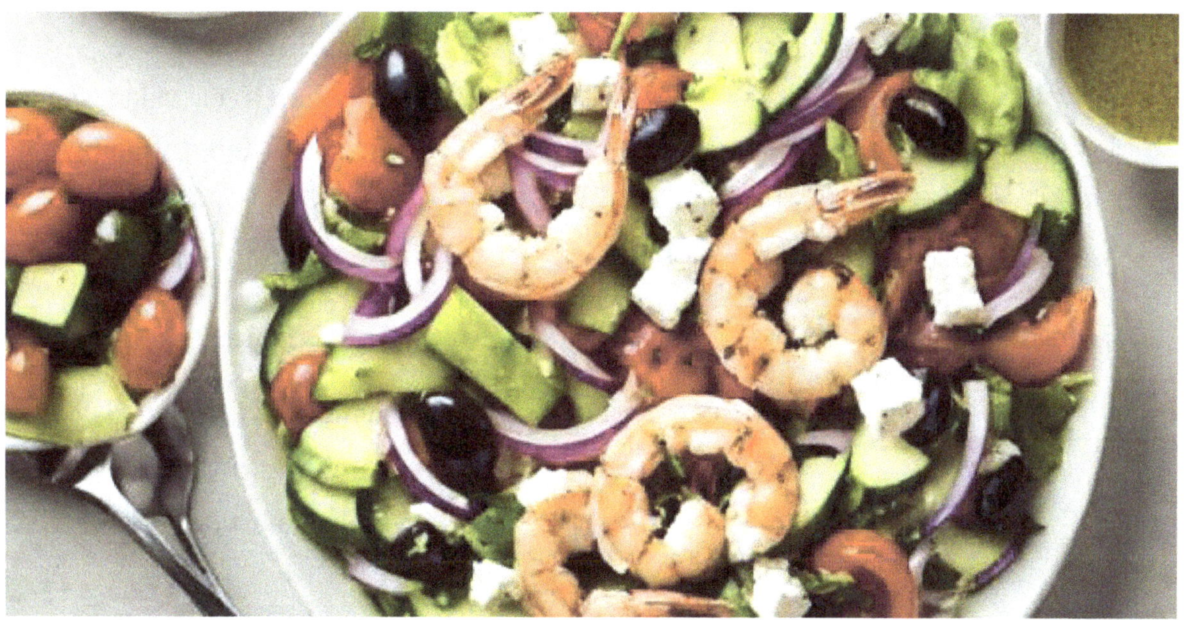

Prep Time: 15 minutes	
Cooking Time: 10 minutes	
Total Time: 25 minutes	
Servings: 4	

Ingredients:

- 1 pound of large shrimp, peeled and deveined
- 1 tablespoon of olive oil
- 1/2 teaspoon of dried oregano
- Salt and pepper to taste
- 8 cups of mixed greens
- 1/2 cup of cherry tomatoes, halved
- 1/2 cup of cucumber, sliced
- 1/4 cup of red onion, sliced
- 1/4 cup of Kalamata olives, pitted
- 1/4 cup of crumbled feta cheese
- 1/4 cup of Greek salad dressing

Directions:

1. Preheat the grill to medium-high heat.
2. In a mixing bowl, toss the shrimp with olive oil, oregano, salt, and pepper.
3. Cook the shrimp on the grill for 2-3 minutes on each side, until they turn pink and opaque.
4. In a large salad bowl, combine the mixed greens, cherry tomatoes, cucumber, red onion, Kalamata olives, and feta cheese.
5. Add the grilled shrimp to the salad.
6. Pour the Greek salad sauce on top of the salad and mix it all together.
7. Serve immediately.

Nutritional Value:

Each serving of this meal contains approximately 200 calories, 20g of protein, and 5g of fiber.

Dinner: Zucchini noodles with turkey meatballs

Prep Time: 15 minutes
Cooking Time: 25 minutes
Total Time: 40 minutes
Servings: 4

Ingredients:

- 1 pound of ground turkey
- 1/2 cup of breadcrumbs
- 1/4 cup of grated Parmesan cheese
- 1/4 cup of chopped fresh parsley
- 1 egg
- 1/2 teaspoon of garlic powder
- Salt and pepper to taste
- 4 medium zucchinis, spiralized
- 2 cups of marinara sauce
- 1/4 cup of shredded mozzarella cheese

Directions:

1. Preheat the oven to 375°F.
2. In a mixing bowl, combine the ground turkey, breadcrumbs, Parmesan cheese, parsley, egg, garlic powder, salt, and pepper.
3. Roll the mixture into 1 1/2-inch meatballs.
4. Place the meatballs on a baking sheet and bake for 20-25 minutes, or until they are cooked through.
5. In a large skillet, heat the marinara sauce over medium heat.
6. Add the zucchini noodles to the skillet and cook for 2-3 minutes, or until they are tender.
7. Divide the zucchini noodles between 4 plates.
8. Top the zucchini noodles with the turkey meatballs.
9. Sprinkle the shredded mozzarella cheese over the meatballs.
10. Serve hot.

Nutritional Value:

Each serving of this meal contains approximately 300 calories, 25g of protein, and 10g of fiber.

Snack: Greek yogurt with honey and almonds:

Prep Time: 5 minutes
Total Time: 5 minutes
Servings: 1

Ingredients:

- 1/2 cup of plain Greek yogurt
- 1 tablespoon of honey
- 1 tablespoon of sliced almonds

Directions:

1. In a tiny bowl, stir the Greek yogurt and honey together.
2. Top with sliced almonds.
3. Enjoy!

Nutritional Value:

Each serving of this snack contains approximately 150 calories, 10g of protein, and 7g of fat

Breakfast: Avocado toast with smoked salmon

Prep Time: 10 minutes
Cooking Time: 5 minutes
Total Time: 15 minutes
Servings: 2

Ingredients:

- 2 slices of whole-grain bread
- 1 ripe avocado
- 4 oz. of smoked salmon
- 1 tablespoon of fresh dill, chopped
- 1 tablespoon of fresh lemon juice
- Salt and pepper to taste

Directions:

1. Toast the bread slices.
2. Use a fork to squish the avocado in a bowl.
3. Add the chopped dill, lemon juice, salt, and pepper to the mashed avocado and mix well.
4. Spread the avocado mixture evenly over the toast slices.
5. Top the avocado toast with smoked salmon.
6. Serve immediately.

Nutritional Value:

Each serving of this meal contains approximately 350 calories, 20g of protein, and 20g of carbohydrates.

Lunch: Tomato and red lentil soup

Prep Time: 10 minutes
Cooking Time: 25 minutes
Total Time: 35 minutes
Servings: 4

Ingredients:

- 1 tablespoon of olive oil
- 1 onion, chopped
- 2 cloves of garlic, minced
- 1 teaspoon of ground cumin
- 1/2 teaspoon of ground coriander
- 1/4 teaspoon of cayenne pepper
- One cup of red lentils, rinsed and drained
- 1 can (14.5 oz.) of diced tomatoes
- 4 cups of vegetable broth
- Salt and pepper to taste

Directions:

1. The olive oil should be heated over medium heat in a big saucepan.
2. Cook the minced garlic and chopped onion in the saucepan until the onion becomes transparent.
3. To the saucepan, add the ground cumin, ground coriander, and cayenne pepper. Cook for one minute.
4. Bring the saucepan to a boil after adding the diced tomatoes, red lentils, and vegetable broth.
5. After lowering the heat, let the lentils simmer for 20 to 25 minutes, or until they become soft.
6. To taste, add more salt and pepper to the soup.
7. Serve hot.

Nutritional Value:

Each serving of this meal contains approximately 250 calories, 15g of protein, and 40g of carbohydrates.

Dinner: Grilled steak with roasted asparagus

Prep Time: 10 minutes
Cooking Time: 20 minutes
Total Time: 30 minutes
Servings: 4

Ingredients:

- 4 ribeye steaks
- 1 lb. of asparagus, trimmed
- 2 tablespoons of olive oil
- 1 tablespoon of garlic powder
- Salt and pepper to taste

Directions:

1. Preheat the grill to medium-high heat.
2. Drizzle the asparagus with olive oil and sprinkle with garlic powder, salt, and pepper.
3. Cook the asparagus on the grill for about 5-7 minutes, or until it is soft when you poke it with a fork.
4. Season the steaks with salt and pepper.
5. Grill the steaks for 3-4 minutes per side, or until they are cooked to your desired level of doneness.
6. Serve the grilled steaks with roasted asparagus.

Nutritional Value:

Each serving of this meal contains approximately 400 calories, 35g of protein, and 5g of carbohydrates

Snack: Sliced cucumber with tzatziki sauce

Prep Time: 10 minutes
Total Time: 10 minutes
Servings: 4

Ingredients:

- 2 medium cucumbers, sliced
- 1 cup of plain Greek yogurt
- 1/2 cup of sour cream
- 1/4 cup of fresh dill, chopped
- 1/4 cup of fresh lemon juice
- 2 cloves of garlic, minced
- Salt and pepper to taste

Directions:

1. In a mixing bowl, whisk together the Greek yogurt, sour cream, chopped dill, lemon juice, minced garlic, salt, and pepper.
2. Arrange the sliced cucumbers on a plate.
3. Drizzle the tzatziki sauce over the cucumbers.
4. Enjoy!

Nutritional Value:

Each serving of this snack contains approximately 100 calories, 5g of protein, and 7g of fat

Breakfast: Gluten-free pancakes with blueberries

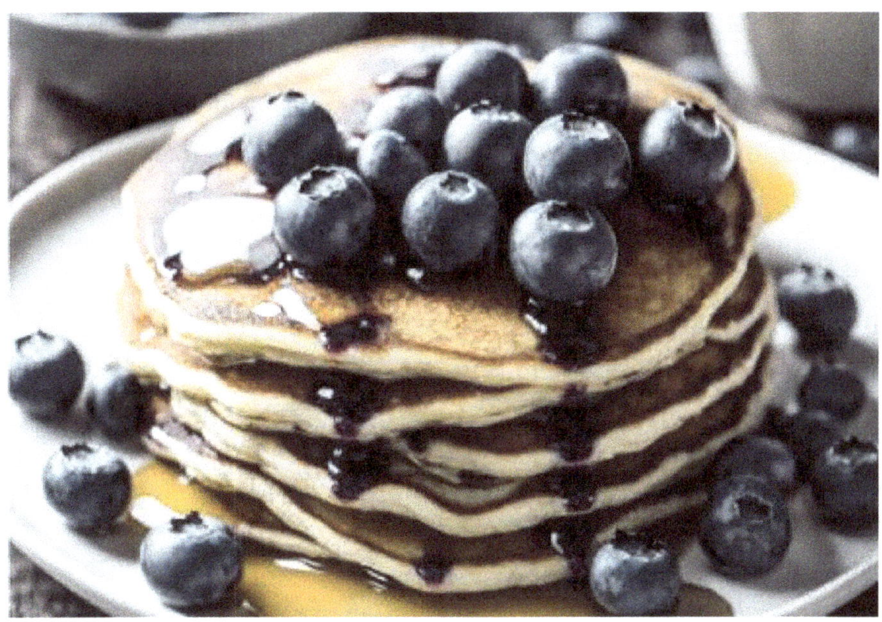

Prep Time: 5 minutes	
Cooking Time: 10 minutes	
Total Time: 15 minutes	
Servings: 4	

Ingredients:

- 1 cup of gluten-free all-purpose flour
- 1 tablespoon of sugar
- 1 teaspoon of baking powder
- 1/2 teaspoon of baking soda
- 1/4 teaspoon of salt
- 1 cup of almond milk
- 1 egg
- 1 tablespoon of vegetable oil
- 1/2 cup of blueberries

Directions:

1. In a mixing bowl, whisk together the gluten-free all-purpose flour, sugar, baking powder, baking soda, and salt.

2. In a separate mixing bowl, whisk together the almond milk, egg, and vegetable oil.

3. Mix the wet ingredients with the dry ingredients gently until they are just mixed together.

4. Then, add the blueberries and mix them in carefully. Next, heat up a special skillet that doesn't stick over medium heat.

5. Pour a small amount of batter onto the skillet for each pancake. Watch for bubbles to appear on the top of the pancake, then flip it over and cook it until it turns a nice golden-brown color.

6. Serve hot with maple syrup or honey.

Nutritional Value:

Each serving of this meal contains approximately 200 calories, 5g of protein, and 30g of carbohydrates1.

Lunch: Mediterranean quinoa salad with grilled chicken

Prep Time: 10 minutes
Cooking Time: 20 minutes
Total Time: 30 minutes
Servings: 4

Ingredients:

- 1 cup of quinoa
- 2 cups of water
- 1/4 cup of olive oil
- 1/4 cup of lemon juice
- 1 teaspoon of honey
- 1/2 teaspoon of salt
- 1/4 teaspoon of black pepper
- 2 cups of cooked chicken, diced
- 1/2 cup of red onion, diced

- 1/2 cup of cucumber, diced
- 1/2 cup of cherry tomatoes, halved
- 1/4 cup of fresh parsley, chopped

Directions:

1. Rinse the quinoa in a fine-mesh strainer and place it in a saucepan with 2 cups of water.
2. Bring the quinoa to a boil, then reduce the heat and simmer for 15-20 minutes, or until the quinoa is tender.
3. In a mixing bowl, whisk together the olive oil, lemon juice, honey, salt, and black pepper.
4. Add the cooked quinoa, chicken, red onion, cucumber, cherry tomatoes, and parsley to the mixing bowl and toss until everything is coated in the dressing.
5. Serve chilled.

Nutritional Value:

Each serving of this meal contains approximately 350 calories, 25g of protein, and 25g of carbohydrates.

Dinner: Baked salmon with roasted vegetables

Prep Time: 10 minutes
Cooking Time: 20 minutes
Total Time: 30 minutes
Servings: 4

Ingredients:

- 4 salmon fillets
- 1 pound of asparagus, trimmed
- 1 pint of cherry tomatoes
- 2 tablespoons of olive oil
- 1 tablespoon of garlic powder
- Salt and pepper to taste

Directions:

1. Preheat the oven to 400°F.
2. In a mixing bowl, toss the asparagus and cherry tomatoes with olive oil, garlic powder, salt, and pepper.
3. Arrange the salmon fillets and vegetables on a baking sheet.
4. Bake for 15 to 20 minutes, or until the veggies are soft and the salmon is cooked through.
5. Serve hot.

Nutritional Value:

Each serving of this meal contains approximately 300 calories, 25g of protein, and 20g of carbohydrates

Snack: Apple slices with almond butter (Refer to Day 1).

Day 6

Breakfast: Greek yogurt with honey and berries

Prep Time: 5 minutes
Total Time: 5 minutes
Servings: 1

Ingredients:

- 1/2 cup of plain Greek yogurt
- Half cup of mixed berries like blueberries, raspberries, strawberries
- 1 tablespoon of honey

Directions:

Mix the Greek yogurt and honey together in a little bowl.

Top with mixed berries.

Enjoy!

Nutritional Value:

Each serving of this breakfast contains approximately 240 calories, 16g of protein, and 44g of carbohydrates.

Lunch: Chickpea and vegetable soup

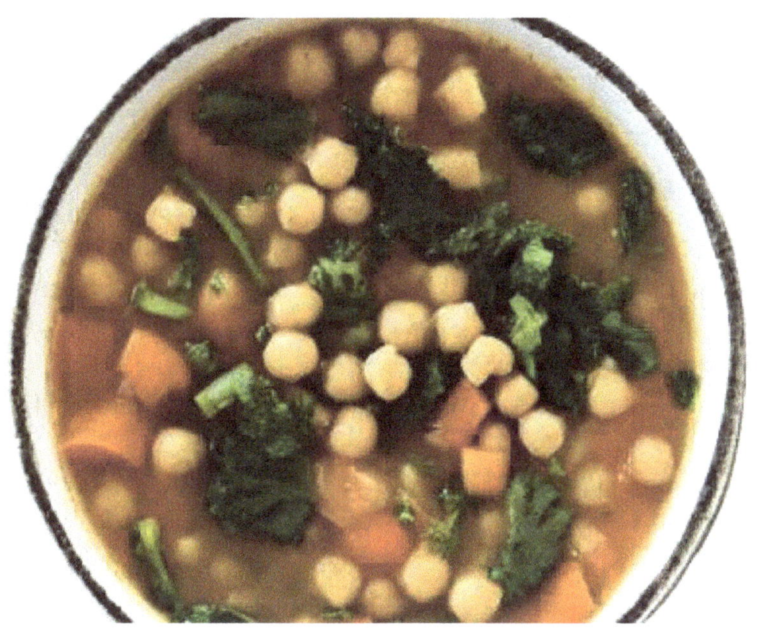

Prep Time: 10 minutes	
Cooking Time: 25 minutes	
Total Time: 35 minutes	
Servings: 4	

Ingredients:

- 1 tablespoon of olive oil
- 1 onion, chopped
- 2 cloves of garlic, minced
- 1 teaspoon of ground cumin
- 1/2 teaspoon of ground coriander
- 1/4 teaspoon of cayenne pepper

- One cup of red lentils, washed and drained
- 1 can (14.5 oz.) of diced tomatoes
- 4 cups of vegetable broth
- Salt and pepper to taste

Directions:

1. In a big pot, warm up the olive oil on medium heat. Put in the cut-up onion and tiny pieces of garlic and cook until the onion looks see-through.
2. Then add the powdered cumin, powdered coriander, and a spicy pepper called cayenne, and cook for just one minute.
3. Next, add the red lentils, diced tomatoes, and vegetable broth to the pot and let it start bubbling. Turn the heat down low and let it cook for about 20 to 25 minutes, until the lentils are soft.
4. Season the soup with salt and pepper to taste.
5. Serve hot.

Nutritional Value:

Each serving of this lunch contains approximately 250 calories, 15g of protein, and 40g of carbohydrates.

Dinner: Grilled chicken with roasted sweet potatoes

Prep Time: 10 minutes
Cooking Time: 20 minutes
Total Time: 30 minutes
Servings: 4

Ingredients:

- 4 boneless, skinless chicken breasts
- 2 large sweet potatoes, peeled and cubed
- 2 tablespoons of olive oil
- 1 teaspoon of garlic powder

- 1 teaspoon of paprika
- 1/2 teaspoon of salt
- 1/4 teaspoon of black pepper

Directions:

1. Preheat the oven to 400°F.
2. In a mixing bowl, whisk together the olive oil, garlic powder, paprika, salt, and black pepper.
3. Add the cubed sweet potatoes to the mixing bowl and toss until they are coated in the seasoning.
4. Place the chicken breasts and sweet potatoes on a baking sheet and bake for 35-40 minutes, or until the chicken is cooked through and the sweet potatoes are tender.
5. Serve hot.

Nutritional Value:

Each serving of this dinner contains approximately 300 calories, 25g of protein, and 20g of carbohydrates.

Snack: Carrots with hummus

Prep Time: 5 minutes
Total Time: 5 minutes
Servings: 1

Ingredients:

- 1 cup of baby carrots
- 3 tablespoons of hummus

Directions:

1. Arrange the baby carrots on a plate.
2. Spoon the hummus into a small bowl.
3. Dip the carrots into the hummus and enjoy!

Nutritional Value:

Each serving of this snack contains approximately 100 calories, 2g of protein, and 10g of carbohydrates

Breakfast: Scrambled eggs mixed with spinach and feta cheese

Prep Time: 5 minutes
Cooking Time: 5 minutes
Total Time: 10 minutes
Servings: 1

Ingredients:

- 3/4 cup of fresh spinach
- 4 large eggs
- 1 tablespoon of butter
- 1 oz. of feta cheese
- 1 pinch of crushed red pepper
- 1 pinch of freshly cracked black pepper
- 1 pinch of salt

Directions:

1. In a big frying pan, let the butter melt on medium heat. Add the spinach and cook until wilted.
2. In a mixing bowl, whisk together the eggs, salt, black pepper, and crushed red pepper.
3. Transfer the beaten eggs to the frying pan and cook until they become firm.
4. Crumble the feta cheese over the eggs and serve hot.

Nutritional Value:

Each serving of this meal contains approximately 240 calories, 16g of protein, and 44g of carbohydrates.

Lunch: Greek salad with grilled shrimp

Prep Time: 15 minutes
Cooking Time: 10 minutes
Total Time: 25 minutes
Servings: 4

Ingredients:

- 1 pound of large shrimp, peeled and deveined
- 1 tablespoon of olive oil
- 1/2 teaspoon of dried oregano
- Salt and pepper to taste
- 8 cups of mixed greens
- 1/2 cup of cherry tomatoes, halved
- 1/2 cup of cucumber, sliced
- 1/4 cup of red onion, sliced
- 1/4 cup of Kalamata olives, pitted
- 1/4 cup of crumbled feta cheese
- 1/4 cup of Greek salad dressing

Directions:

1. Preheat the grill to medium-high heat.
2. In a mixing bowl, toss the shrimp with olive oil, oregano, salt, and pepper.
3. Cook the shrimp on the grill for about 2-3 minutes on each side, or until they turn pink and you can't see through them.
4. In a large salad bowl, combine the mixed greens, cherry tomatoes, cucumber, red onion, Kalamata olives, and feta cheese.
5. Add the grilled shrimp to the salad.
6. Pour the Greek salad dressing on top of the salad and mix it together.
7. Serve immediately.

Nutritional Value:

Each serving of this meal contains approximately 200 calories, 20g of protein, and 5g of fiber.

Dinner: Zucchini noodles with turkey meatballs

Prep Time: 15 minutes
Cooking Time: 25 minutes
Total Time: 40 minutes
Servings: 4

Ingredients:

- 1 pound of ground turkey
- 1/2 cup of breadcrumbs
- 1/4 cup of grated Parmesan cheese
- 1/4 cup of chopped fresh parsley
- 1 egg
- 1/2 teaspoon of garlic powder
- Salt and pepper to taste
- 4 medium zucchinis, spiralized
- 2 cups of marinara sauce
- 1/4 cup of shredded mozzarella cheese

Directions:

1. Preheat the oven to 375°F.
2. In a mixing bowl, combine the ground turkey, breadcrumbs, Parmesan cheese, parsley, egg, garlic powder, salt, and pepper.
3. Roll the mixture into 1 1/2-inch meatballs.
4. Place the meatballs on a baking sheet and bake for 20-25 minutes, or until they are cooked through.
5. In a large skillet, heat the marinara sauce over medium heat.
6. Add the zucchini noodles to the skillet and cook for 2-3 minutes, or until they are tender.

7. Divide the zucchini noodles between 4 plates.
8. Top the zucchini noodles with the turkey meatballs.
9. Sprinkle the shredded mozzarella cheese over the meatballs.
10. Serve hot.

Nutritional Value:

Each serving of this meal contains approximately 300 calories, 25g of protein, and 10g of fiber.

Snack: Greek yogurt with honey and almonds (Refer to Day 3).

Happy Cooking!